My Training Journal

A comprehensive journal for tracking fitness
training and nutritional intake.

Aaron R. Tews, BSc Kinesiology

Order this book online at www.trafford.com
or email orders@trafford.com

Most Trafford titles are also available at major online book retailers.

Printed in the United States of America.

ISBN: 978-1-4251-7961-8 (sc)

Trafford rev. 02/23/2012

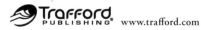 www.trafford.com

North America & international
toll-free: 1 888 232 4444 (USA & Canada)
phone: 250 383 6864 ♦ fax: 812 355 4082

The enclosed information has been reviewed and every effort has been made to make the resource as accurate as possible.

This resource should not be used as a substitute for professional, medical or recreational counseling or instruction. Everyone should consult the appropriate professional for guidance before starting any exercise program. The author disclaims any liability from loss, injury, or damage personal or otherwise, resulting from the information in this book.

Do you have a question or comment or would like to report an error?
Email: **info@vipfitness.ca**

Also, be sure to check out: **vipfitness.ca**

Preface

I am not the ideal age, the ideal weight, nor the ideal shape.
There are things that will keep me from a goal of being the Hollywood ideal.
Genetics, age, health, and body type just to name a few.
But I can be a healthier, happier, fitter person by having exercise as part of my life.
No matter what my physical, mental, social or financial limitations,
I can work towards a better quality of life.

Aaron Tews, BSc. Kinesiology, CPT, RK, FMS, BCRPA TFL

Aaron graduated from the University of Victoria with a BSc. Kinesiology in 1993 and started his company VIP (Vancouver Island Professional) Fitness. His certification, memberships and accomplishments include: Practicing member of the BCAK (British Columbia Association of Kinesiologists) since 1995; Member of the Board of Directors of the BCAK, Member of BCRPA as a recognized Trainer of Trainers for the Fitness Theory course, the Strength Training Specialty Module and the Personal Trainer courses since the mid-90's; and Certified instructor for the CPAFLA (Canadian Physical Activity, Fitness & Lifestyle Appraisal) course. In 2010, he completed Gray Cook's Functional Movement Screen (FMS) Certification. Aaron has published a book on resistance training called "A Professional Guide to Resistance Training (2005)." He also had the first BCRPA-recognized correspondence course for the Strength Training Specialty Module in the province of British Columbia.

Aaron also owns a rehabilitation / physical culture studio in Vancouver (Kitsilano), BC called KINESIOLOGISTS dot CA (InFOCUS Wellness Inc. dba).

I would like to acknowledge the following people for their encouragement over the years as I ran around teaching others about fitness and spending way to many hours in front of my computer.

> **Gillian Tews** - without your love and support, this journal would not have been possible. Thank you!

> **Christina Truscott** - a friend and professional colleague. Thanks for all your assistance over the years. Here is to many more!

> **Stephen Robinson** - your support and encouragement to complete this journal and all other projects has been invaluable. Your feedback has been especially important. Here is to another 15 years of training and friendship!

> **Steve McMinn & Graeme Lehman** - who reintroduced me to the excitement and energy our industry holds.

Thanks to you all.

Table of Contents

General Theory

The following information has been used with permission from the book *"A Professional Guide to Resistance Training"* written by Aaron Tews and published in 2005.

Benefits of Training

Over the years there has been a substantial amount of information to both support and discredit regular fitness training (cardiovascular, resistance, stretching) to improve and maintain one's health profile. Listed below are several benefits and potential hazards associated with training. The potential benefits include , but are not limited to:

- Increased body awareness.
- Increased sense of vitality.
- Refreshes the mind.
- Reduced mental fatigue.
- Development and maintenance of muscular strength, muscular mass, muscular endurance and muscular power.
- Increased bone density and bone mass.
- Increased strength of connective tissue.
- Prevention of age associated decline in muscle mass and strength.
- May result in decreased resting heart rate, but this is dependent on overall training intensity.
- Prevention of age associated decline in metabolic rate.
- Decreased systolic and diastolic blood pressure levels.
- Provides an enjoyable time for socializing with friends or family.

Guidelines for Sensible Training

Establish training goals. Be aware of what is to be accomplished through the training program - lose weight, improve muscular strength, muscular power and/or muscular endurance, get huge, rehabilitate an injury or improve cardiovascular fitness.

Engage in an effective and efficient training program. Ensure the program is based upon scientific principles, time and energy are not wasted, exercises are appropriate, and training equipment (modality) is appropriate for ability and knowledge.

Safety must be of utmost concern. Perform exercises that do not hurt. Be sure to have medical clearance before beginning an exercise program. When unsure, err on the side of caution. Perform exercises properly - technique, technique, technique!

Have a fitness assessment prior to beginning a training program. An assessment sets your fitness baseline and determines weak and strong areas. Do not have assessments too regularly to avoid discouragement when dramatic results slow down.

Aim for total fitness. Strength training is only one area of overall fitness. Remember to train for cardiovascular fitness, muscular strength, muscular endurance, and flexibility. Be well balanced!

Develop sound nutritional habits. If you do not eat sensibly, results will be slow. Remember that you are what you eat!

Avoid over-training. Too much too soon makes exercise uncomfortable and decreases interest. Over-training decreases performance and slows results. Exercise should be enjoyable and not feel like a contest.

Keep a training diary. A detailed strength training diary will help evaluate program effectiveness. In times of plateaus, the diary may serve as an excellent motivator!

Train for the health of it! If driving to the gym across town takes up lots of time and raises stress levels think about exercising at home. Exercise for the health benefits. Make exercise a part of your lifestyle.

Ensure your training program is enjoyable. A boring strength training program results in, well, boredom! A professionally designed program is creative, maintains interest levels, and is safe and effective.

- Reduction of stress levels.
- Combined with healthy eating, may improve self image.
- Associated with modest improvements in cholesterol profiles.
- Muscular strength increases.
- Improvements in cardiovascular fitness through strength training and substantial improvement through circuit training.
- Modest decrease in body fat through strength training and a substantial decrease through circuit training and cardiovascular training.

The potential health risks include , but are not limited to:

- Possibility of decreased flexibility.
- Increased risk of injury to joints and muscles due to improper technique, broken equipment or overtraining.

Four Essential Phases of Every Training Session

A well designed program should always incorporate the four phases of a training session.

Warm-up Phase. It is not uncommon to neglect the warm-up phase of a training session. A warm-up should last between 5 and 15 minutes to raise the body temperature. The intensity of the warm-up should be increased gradually to avoid muscular fatigue. A warm-up should incorporate the muscle groups that will be used during the workout. The benefits of a good warm-up include:

- Stimulates the release of synovial fluid (reduces joint friction and increases joint mobility).
- Should simulate the movements incorporated in a workout, which enhances neuromuscular coordination.
- Increases body temperature and warms up the muscles.
- Gradually raises the heart rate.
- Blood vessels dilate to more readily supply blood / oxygen / nutrients to the working muscles.
- Increases a joints range of motion. This may alleviate tension in muscles and connective tissue; and may also reduce the risk of strains and sprains.

Stretching Phase. The stretching phase follows the warm-up phase. It is more effective to stretch after a warm-up than prior to it. This phase should last about 5 minutes to prevent the body from returning to its pre-warmed state.

Three - Workout Phase. This phase is considered the body or bulk of an exercise session. All workouts are not created equal. Practice is required to design effective and efficient workout programs. The workout may be comprised of weight training, cardiovascular training or both.

Cool-down Phase. The cool-down is important because it may reduce the uncomfortable effects associated with delayed onset muscle soreness and speeds up the removal of waste products from active cells. The cool-down should consist of mild aerobic exercise and easy stretching because fatigued muscles are susceptible to strains. In summary, it prepares the body for rest.

Skeletal Muscle

Skeletal muscles, provide movement to body limbs and the torso. The muscles required to generate the forces necessary to move weights and bars in the gym usually work in groups rather than separately.

Muscle Actions

The terminology used to describe muscle contractions are below.

Concentric Muscle Action - muscle action in which the muscle is shortening under its own power. An example is the biceps muscles during the lifting phase of the barbell biceps curls.

Eccentric Muscle Action - muscle action in where the muscle resists as it is forced to lengthen. An example is the pectoral muscle during the lowering phase of the bench press. This is the most important phase when weight training so focus most effort on resisting gravity for maximum results.

Isometric Muscle Action - muscle action in which the muscle attempts to contract against a fixed limit or resistance. An example is pushing against a wall.

Isotonic Muscle Action - muscle action in which the muscle shortens against a constant tension. This term is applied to free-weight exercises and fixed resistance machines because the load remains constant throughout the range of motion.

Isokinetic Muscle Action - muscle action in which a muscle shortens against a resistance that moves at a constant velocity. This is often used in a rehabilitation setting and involves sophisticated computer assisted devices.

Common Exercise-Attributed Muscular Soreness

Discomfort and soreness experienced during or after an exercise session is believed in part to be caused by chemical substances released by damaged tissues. The chemical substances stimulate sensory receptors and the sensation of pain is a result. Although the occurrence of muscular soreness is a common event related to exercise, the true cause remains unknown.

In general, muscular discomfort related to physical activity can be divided into two categories - acute onset muscular soreness (AOMS) and delayed onset muscular soreness (DOMS).

Acute Onset Muscular Soreness (AOMS). Although the true cause of AOMS is unknown, onset occurs during and immediately following an exercise and is thought to be associated with a lack of blood flow to active tissues The degree of soreness varies between individuals because of different pain thresholds.

Delayed Onset Muscular Soreness (DOMS). DOMS pain is associated with damage to the muscle fibre brought on primarily during the performance of slow eccentric muscle actions or unaccustomed activity. DOMS may indicate a few rest days are required to allow the body to repair. To minimize muscular soreness during the first few weeks of a weight training program, perform 1-2 sets and 15+ repetitions, focusing on technique rather than the weight. After the first two weeks, the volume and intensity of training can be gradually

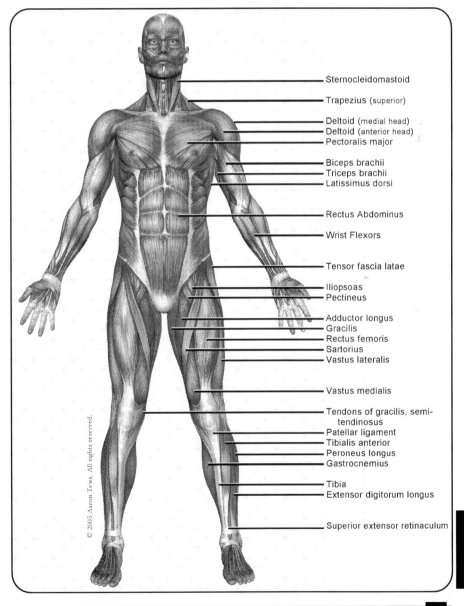

Sternocleidomastoid

Trapezius (superior)

Deltoid (medial head)
Deltoid (anterior head)
Pectoralis major

Biceps brachii
Triceps brachii
Latissimus dorsi

Rectus Abdominus

Wrist Flexors

Tensor fascia latae

Iliopsoas
Pectineus

Adductor longus
Gracilis
Rectus femoris
Sartorius
Vastus lateralis

Vastus medialis

Tendons of gracilis, semi-
tendinosus
Patellar ligament
Tibialis anterior
Peroneus longus
Gastrocnemius

Tibia
Extensor digitorum longus

Superior extensor retinaculum

increased without significant increases in DOMS. With cardiovascular training, be sure to increase the intensity and duration slowly. Several measures used to avoid DOMS include a good stretching session prior to, and after a workout, a gradual progression in intensity and the ingestion of Vitamin C.

Stretching

Stretching is frequently neglected. The neglect is often due to the time commitment necessary to improve beyond a basic level of flexibility. A common

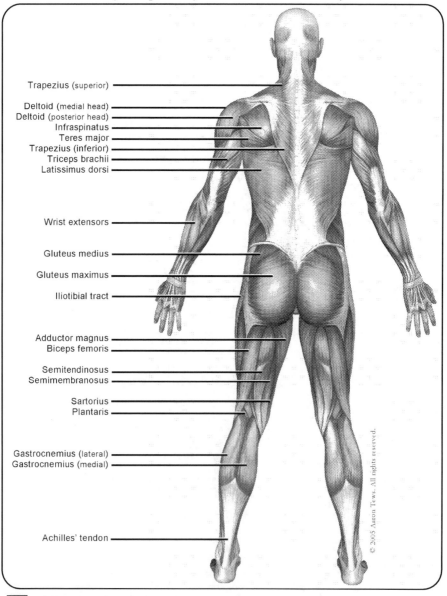

Trapezius (superior)
Deltoid (medial head)
Deltoid (posterior head)
Infraspinatus
Teres major
Trapezius (inferior)
Triceps brachii
Latissimus dorsi

Wrist extensors

Gluteus medius

Gluteus maximus

Iliotibial tract

Adductor magnus
Biceps femoris

Semitendinosus
Semimembranosus

Sartorius
Plantaris

Gastrocnemius (lateral)
Gastrocnemius (medial)

Achilles' tendon

misnomer is that strength training decreases flexibility. Often, a decrease in flexibility is due to an inadequate or non-participation in a stretching program. Some bodybuilders are extremely flexible because of their rigorous stretching program.

Why stretch? Although scientific research has not proven that stretching and being flexible help prevent injury, there are many non-scientific reasons for including stretching in a fitness program. Several reasons for stretching are that it *may* assist in preventing muscle strains, is known to promote good circulation, prepares the body for exercise (stimulates the muscles that are going to be used during the activity), develops a personal body awareness (focuses attention on specific areas of the body), increases range of motion (thus may increase force development), reduces muscle tension, it just *feels* good for some, and helps improve coordination by allowing for freer and easier movement.

Flexibility appears to decrease with age and is attributed primarily to decreased movement rather than age related problems. An age related decrease in flexibility is not permanent and can often be recovered. Past injury and the subsequent build-up of scar tissue may also decrease flexibility, but stretching actually aids in decreasing the buildup of scar tissue. Lastly, some people are genetically blessed with greater flexibility than others.

Flexibility Development

As with other fitness components, stretching programs follow the FITT principle. The *frequency* of stretching may be 2 to 5 times per week, but everyday is great; *intensity* - stretch to the point of mild discomfort and then ease off slightly; *time* - start with holding the stretch a minimum of 10 seconds and then increase by 5 second increments to a maximum of 90 seconds for 1-4 sets; *type* - static and include all the major muscle groups.

Basic Stretching Technique

The following are guidelines for safe stretching programs:

- Do not stretch too far, especially at the beginning of a session and the start of a stretching program.
- Hold stretch in a comfortable position, just below the point of discomfort; the amount of discomfort should decrease as the stretch is held.
- Breathing should be deep, slow, and natural. Avoid stretching to the point where breathing is compromised - especially if you are overweight.
- Exhale while positioning into the stretch.
- Never continue a stretch if it is painful.
- Concentrate on postural alignment.
- Do not bounce.
- Focus on the area being stretched.
- Do not try to be flexible. Learn to stretch properly first and flexibility will follow.
- Do not wear restrictive clothing.
- It is best to warm up prior to stretching.
- Adjust to the changing body - everyday the body will feel slightly different and will respond to stretching differently.

- Be aware of head, shoulder, and lower back alignment during a stretch.

There are an infinite number of stretches that could be performed before each workout. However, depending on time factors and goals, the actual stretches performed will be dictated by the instructor.

Cardiovascular Training

Intensity of Exercise

When the terms 'target heart zone,' 'target heart rate,' and 'exercise intensity' are used, it is often to describe the safe range the heart should beat per minute during an exercise session. It is possible to train in the target heart rate zone during a resistance training session by circuit training, dynamic heart action or hydra-gym fitness programs.

In order to calculate your target heart rate, one of several mathematical formulas may be used. Most methods use a percentage of a persons maximum heart rate and/ or the resting heart rate. An individual's *maximum heart rate* (MHR) is calculated by subtracting their age from 220. A resting heart rate is usually taken in the lying position (radially or at the carotid artery) just before getting up in the morning (number of beats in one minute).

There are several methods used to determine training workload and intensity during cardiovascular exercise.

Standard Target Zone Method. This method calculates an exercise intensity based on 70% to 85% of the maximum heart rate.

Target Zone = [(220-age) x (60%) and (85%)]

Karvonen Formula or Heart Rate Reserve Method (HRR). This method is considered more accurate than the Standard Target Zone method because it incorporates a person's resting heart rate (RHR) into the equation. This equation calculates the target heart rate range as follows:

Target Zone = [((220 - age) - RHR) x (60%) and (85%)] + RHR

If fat loss is your primary focus, the recommended training zone is 60 to 70% of MHR. Training in this zone is also great for beginners unable to sustain higher training levels, those wanting to train for longer periods of time (20 minutes +) and those who find working at a lower intensity more comfortable.

The benefits of training between 70 to 90% of MHR are a more intense and shorter workout, increased stress placed upon the cardiovascular system, increased metabolic rate post exercise, and an increase in anaerobic threshold tolerance. Training in this zone is not recommended for beginners, but recommended for moderately fit to fit individuals.

Weight Training

Determining Set and Repetition Ranges

Sets & Repetitions

The aim of resistance training is to progressively overload the muscle. When the training load exceeds general daily requirements, the body responds by overcompensating, thereby equipping the muscle to handle increased load. These changes allow the person to perform exercises with greater ease. In general, a beginner would start with higher repetitions (15+) and a low number of sets (1 to 2).

There is no rule as to the number of sets a person should perform. Rather, it depends on your ability, fitness levels, personal goals and skill development.

The number of repetitions performed is the key to training success. As with sets, there is no 'rule' for determining the number of repetitions. However, age, gender, ability level, desire, training background, training goal, and training volume are several variables that influence the number of repetitions a program planner may design the program around.

The benefits associated with the number of repetitions performed is the point of complete muscular fatigue (cannot perform even one more repetition without sacrificing technique). The point of total muscular failure varies between individuals, from one workout session to another and from one week to the next. However, training consistently to total muscular fatigue is directly related to greater results. It is very difficult to train maximally *every* session, as a rule of thumb, one maximal training period per week, per muscle group is sufficient.

The speed of each repetition also has an impact on training gains. As a rule of thumb, the speed of each repetition should be slow and controlled. This varies anywhere from 2 - 6+ seconds on the lowering phase and 2 - 6+ seconds on the lifting phase. In addition, you should avoid pausing between each repetition during a set.

Determining the length of your rest periods (time between sets)

When deciding on the length of rest between sets it should be based on the time you have to exercise. With a one minute rest between sets, a program with 3 sets for 8 exercises has almost 25 minutes of rest! If you decrease the rest period to 30 seconds, your program would take 12 minutes less to perform. It may take you several weeks of training before being capable of a 30 second rest interval between sets if your cardiovascular conditioning is poor.

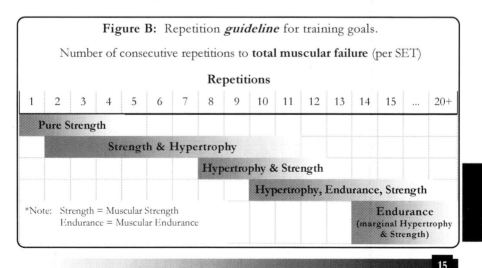

Figure B: Repetition *guideline* for training goals.

Number of consecutive repetitions to **total muscular failure** (per SET)

Repetitions

1	2	3	4	5	6	7	8	9	10	11	12	13	14	15	...	20+

Pure Strength

Strength & Hypertrophy

Hypertrophy & Strength

Hypertrophy, Endurance, Strength

Endurance (marginal Hypertrophy & Strength)

*Note: Strength = Muscular Strength
Endurance = Muscular Endurance

A program with little or no rest between sets is called circuit training and is very common for those with limited amounts of time for training.

Determining your program's duration

A program may last between one day and 6 weeks, but the same program should never last longer than 8 weeks. Resistance training requires continual modification to be effective.

Adding variety to your training program

There are an infinite ways of making a program more interesting and challenging. Below is a list of ways to spice up a program.

Multiple Sets: More than 1 set (usually 2 to 5) of each exercise is performed before proceeding to the next exercise. For example, 3 sets of flat bench barbell chest press of 12-15 repetitions.

Super Set: Two exercises are performed in succession without rest. After the second exercise is completed, rest before beginning the next super set.

Super Tri-Sets: Similar to super sets, but three exercises follow one another.

Ascending Sets: Perform multiple sets, but the load is increased and the number of repetitions decreased with each succeeding set. A rest period is usually included between each set.

Descending Sets: Perform multiple sets, but the load is decreased and the number of repetitions increases with each succeeding set. A rest period is usually included between each set.

Pyramid Sets: Perform multiple sets combining ascending and descending sets. A rest period is usually included between each set.

Staggered Sets: With staggered sets, also referred to as alternating sets, one muscle group is exercised between other exercises in a program. It is often incorporated for a muscle group that a participant does not like to train, or forgets to train.

21's: This method is designed to totally fatigue a particular muscle or group. With this method, 7 repetitions are performed in the lower half of the range of motion, 7 repetitions in the upper half of the range of motion and 7 repetitions are performed using the full range of motion for a total of 21 repetitions.

Strip Sets / Running the Rack: Usually, a strip set is performed as the last set of a particular exercise. For an exercise with 4 sets, on the fourth set use a load which will allow you to perform 4 to 6 repetitions. When you are unable to perform any more repetitions, decrease the weight. Again, when the muscle is fully fatigued at that weight, remove more weight and so on until as many strips as desired have been performed. The key to an effective strip set is minimal rest during the stripping. When dumbbells are used for a strip set, simply 'run the rack.' Strip sets should be performed once per exercise and once per muscle group.

I Go - You Go: This method requires a training partner and is designed to push training boundaries. With this method, one person performs as many repetitions as possible with an exercise. After the initial set is completed, the second person performs the same exercise immediately. This process is repeated until the predetermined number of sets are completed.

Circuit Training: With circuit training, all exercises are completed once before any exercise is repeated. Rest periods are virtually eliminated (except the amount of time needed to change stations). The object is to perform as many *controlled* repetitions as possible during a specific period of time - usually 30 seconds. Circuit training programs can be designed for exercise machines, free weights (although not common), and body weight exercises. Circuit training is highly effective for those with limited time to train. The benefits of circuit training are improved cardiovascular conditioning, muscular endurance, and muscular strength.

Split Routine: By designing a split routine, several exercises per body part can be performed each session. Split routines can be half-day, 2-day, 3-day, 4-day, 5-day or more. The most common is the 2-day split where the upper body is worked one day and the lower body the next.

Split Program: Split programs are not to be confused with split routines. Split programs train the whole body every workout, but different exercises are used. This type of program should not be performed everyday so as to give the body a rest. An example of a split program is:

Principles of SMART Training

Progressive Overload Principle: When applied to resistance training, this principle is defined as a gradual and systematic increase in the stress or demand placed upon the neuromuscular system. Examples of the progressive overload principle applied to resistance training would be increasing resistance, decreasing rest periods between sets and / or increasing the number of exercises per workout.

Specificity of Overload Principle (SAID): This principle states that the body will adapt specifically to meet new demands placed upon it and the training effect is specific in speed, resistance, duration, muscle groups and joint actions. This principle is often referred to as the SAID Principle (Specific Adaptation to Imposed Demands).

Rest Principle: In response to a training session, the body will show some breakdown and requires rest to rebuild greater than the pre-training level. The length of rest required for the rebuilding process will vary depending on the type of training (e.g. muscular endurance, muscular power) and the intensity. Without adequate rest, the problems associated with overtraining are inevitable.

Priority Principle: Priority is placed on muscle groups needing the greatest improvement. Exercises for the weakest muscle or muscle group are placed at the beginning of the program when energy levels are high. For example, if the biceps are the weak point, ensure they are exercised before working the back muscles.

Program Design Guidelines

Weight Training

Muscle Mass / Hypertrophy Training (increasing muscle size)

Increasing muscle size is dependent upon maximizing resistance training efficiency and effectiveness while minimizing injury and overtraining. This is best accomplished following a sensible training program and understanding how the body adapts to training. A program must be designed a certain way to stimulate the process of protein synthesis for muscle growth.

Muscle Tension

Tension on a muscle stimulates protein synthesis. Tension demand on a muscle is impacted by the speed of the concentric and eccentric phases of a particular exercise. The phrase 'Time At Tension' is important to remember.

Time at tension is linked to repetition and set ranges. Muscle size increase occurs primarily within the 3+ sets of 6 to 12 repetitions range. Pausing between each repetition is ineffective and will not maximize protein synthesis.

Type of Muscle Actions Involved

Increasing the size of muscle fibres is also dependent upon the type of muscle actions involved. A study by McCall et al. (1996) confirmed the importance of controlled lifting and lowering phases of each repetition. A common error in the gym is to concentrate on the lifting phase of an exercise and not the lowering phase. It is suggested that a 3 second concentric and 3 second eccentric count be used when performing all repetitions.

Hormonal Status

Protein synthesis is influenced by certain hormones in our bodies. Three hormones which influence protein synthesis significantly are testosterone, growth hormone (GH) and insulin-like growth factors. Each hormone influences the muscle fibres nuclei to increase production of muscle tissue. Increased levels of muscle tissue production is known as anabolism. Testosterone (anabolic hormone) is known to be the primary hormone involved in muscle anabolism.

Other hormones cause the breakdown of muscle protein. The adrenal glands, located on the top of the kidneys, produce hormones known as corticosteroids such as cortisol (catabolic hormone), during times of increased physical stress. The breakdown of muscle tissue due to increased levels of cortisol is known as catabolism. After extremely intense workouts or during periods of overtraining, the amount of anabolic to catabolic hormones decreases, forcing the body into a catabolic state.

Nutritional Considerations

Your nutritional status is important for ensuring muscle mass increases. Amino acids are important for the process of anabolism. Most people have enough protein in their diets. However, during heavy training protein intake may fall below the body's requirements resulting in decreased muscle synthesis. If a person is in a negative caloric intake state (caloric expenditure is greater than caloric intake) then the body may stop synthesizing muscle tissue or actually begin to break down its structural protein. So, it is important to be taking in appropriate amounts of protein, carbohydrates and fats to maximize muscle protein synthesis.

'Strength' Training

Strength training refers to the sole purpose of improving muscle strength. The purpose of training strictly for muscular strength is to improve the ability of the brain to send neural signals to muscles involved in an exercise.

Increasing muscle strength without increasing muscle mass is beneficial to athletes involved in activities such as gymnastics or where there are weight categories such as wrestling and weightlifting.

Speed-Strength (Power) Training

Without getting too technical, speed-strength training is the process of applying speed of execution to improve athletic performance. It is also known as power training and incorporates explosive movements with muscular strength. In certain sports, strength is important, but the ability to use strength quickly (speed) is even more important.

Training for speed is difficult with free weights or machines and is usually done with hydra gym or Kaiser fitness equipment. Speed training with free weights should not be attempted because the weights are affected by momentum.

Sports Specific Training

To improve performance, athletes resistance train. Sprinters, long-distance runners, gymnasts, volleyball players, swimmers and boxers all have resistance training programs designed to improve their athletic performance. Designing programs for specific sports is beyond the scope of this journal, but many books and websites have detailed information on sport specific training programs .

Interval Training

Interval training consists of repeated intervals of relatively high intensity events such as jogging or running or sprinting incongruent with relatively light intensity events such as walking. The light interval would be done in range from 50-70% of your maximum heart rate while the hard interval training would range from 85%-100% of your maximum heart rate. Interval training is highly desirable and beneficial for anti-aging purposes if provided as a break in routine and to train your body to adapt to different stresses from different activity. Interval training also causes a rise in our base metabolic rate (BMR) after the exercise has ended. This increase has effectively cause a body to burn more calorie and keep our fat off. It is, therefore, especially good if you want to reduce the fat in your body.

Safety Considerations & Injury Prevention

Some people are genetically prone or predisposed to injuries through the process of resistance training. For example, predisposition may manifest itself via personality trait (Type A) or joint structure (elbows which hyperextend). The four areas commonly prone to injury, known as the "Famous 4" are the shoulders, neck, lower back and knees. Other areas susceptible to injury are the elbows and wrists. Below is a list of exercises which may aggravate specific areas. Note: *this information should never be used as a substitute for medical help*.

Shoulders

- Exercises for the rotator cuff muscles using heavy loads.
- Failing to exercise the deltoids for balance (anterior, medial, and posterior heads).
- Lat pulldown - behind the neck.
- Locking out the elbows during barbell bench presses (flat, incline, or decline).
- Dumbbell pullovers.
- Improperly adjusted pectoral flye machines.
- Upright rows, especially with internal rotation.
- Straight arms while performing dumbbell medial, anterior or posterior raises.

Neck

- Raising the head off the bench while performing exercises such as barbell chest press.
- Neck strengthening exercises.
- Hyper-extending the neck to watch form in a mirror.
- Incorrectly supporting the barbell on the shoulders during squats.

Lower Back

- Most exercises can affect the lower back if performed incorrectly.
- High risk exercises such as the squat, cleans, or modified deadlifts that require significant training experience and practice.
- Contraindicated exercises such as deadlifts or goodmornings.
- Rotation of the spine against a resistance (i.e. torso twist machine).
- Lifting the hips off the bench during heavy, prone hamstrings curls.
- Picking up weights (plates, dumbbells) with improper lifting techniques or body mechanics.

Knees

- Low cable adductor or abductor pulls.
- Improperly adjusted leg extension machine or using too much weight.
- Squats or incline leg press with toes pointed inward.
- Failing to align the hips, knees, and ankles during the squat, leg press, leg extension, etc.
- Full extension or hyper-extension of the knees.
- Deep squats (knee angle less than 90 degrees).

Elbows

- Locking out the elbow during any exercise or stretch.
- Deep triceps dips.
- Certain preacher curl benches.

Wrists

- Failing to stabilize your wrist(s) while performing certain exercises (e.g. triceps pressdowns).
- Narrow or wide grip bench press.

- Narrow or wide grip barbell curls.
- Heavy wrist curls and wrist extensions.

Injury Prevention Techniques

The best medicine is injury prevention. There are several ways to help minimize the chances of injuring yourself or others while resistance training. Several ideas are listed below.

- Warm-up properly - follow proper warm-up guidelines.
- Stretch the muscles that will be trained, including stabilizers, where possible.
- Follow safe exercise technique and never perform exercises you are unsure about - ask a qualified trainer for help.
- Know your limits - do not train beyond your capability.
- Strive for muscle balance. This includes opposing muscle groups (quadriceps and hamstrings) and body areas (upper and lower body).
- Ensure all major muscle groups are exercised regularly.
- Breathe correctly - exhale on exertion.
- Control the weight - do not let the weight control you!
- Avoid using momentum and ballistic movements with stretching and exercises.
- Avoid rapid weight increases in short periods of time - especially for beginners. Increase repetitions before increasing weight.
- Ensure machines are adjusted correctly. If a machine cannot be adjusted to feel comfortable, avoid performing the exercise.
- Always assume correct postural alignment for any exercise execution while standing - feet shoulder width apart, neutral pelvis tilt (midway between an anterior and a posterior pelvic tilt), slight lumbar curve, knees slightly bent, scapulae slightly retracted and depressed (chest out), abdominal muscles tight (specifically the transversus abdominus and pelvic floor), eyes looking straight ahead, ears aligned over the shoulders, shoulders aligned over the hips, hips aligned over the knees and the knees aligned over the ankles.
- Avoid over-training and overstraining.
- Always be conscious of the position and tension on the spinal column.
- Compete with yourself, not others. This is very hard for some people to do. Do what you can and do not feel pressure to improve quickly. Exercise for the health of it!
- Be sure to perform an adequate cool-down.

Weightlifting Belts

The purpose of a weightlifting belt is to provide support for the lower back. By forming a firm conduit-like structure that both reduces flexion of the spine and increases intra-abdominal pressure (IAP), a weight belt may actually decrease the compressive forces on the lumbar discs.

IAP reduces the need for contraction of the lower back muscles (e.g. erector spinae muscles) when performing a lift. Erector spinae muscles tend to compress the spinal discs, thus the reduction in activity of these muscles when wearing a belt is said to reduce the chance of compressive injury to the spinal discs.

Some weight lifters have expressed that they *feel* more comfortable and safe while wearing a belt, thus weightlifting belts may provide psychological support. However, the potential dangers and limitations of weight belts should also be considered before investing in this device. Potential dangers and limitations of a weightlifting belt are:

- May increase blood pressure and heart rate.
- Limits strengthening of abdominal and lower back muscles.
- May force a lifter to become physically and psychologically dependent.
- Compensates for weak abdominal muscles.

Using a weightlifting belt during rest and exercise tends to increase blood pressure and heart rate. High IAP and intra-thoracic pressures created by the belt may cause vasoconstriction of vessels in the abdominal and thoracic cavities. Blood flow back to the heart may be hindered, thus causing a rise in blood pressure and heart rate. Since blood pressure and heart rate increase normally during exercise, additional elevation caused by the pressure of the weight-belt may be dangerous. An individual with a compromised cardiovascular system (e.g. high blood pressure) may be at a greater health risk when using a weight-belt.

A weight-belt may actually limit the progressive strengthening of the stabilizer muscles as lifting loads increase. EMG (electromyogram) studies have shown that activity of the erector spinae, external oblique, and rectus abdominus muscles was decreased when a weight-belt was worn. Over the long term, these particular stabilizer muscles may actually weaken if the belt is worn excessively.

A lifter may become physically and psychologically dependent on the belt for support. A lifter who wears a belt routinely for most exercises should be cautious when lifting without a belt. Psychologically, the lifter may not feel confident or safe without the belt and may feel the need to wear a belt for most exercises. In many sports and daily activities, varying dynamic eccentric and concentric muscle actions are performed by these postural muscles without a weight-belt. It would seem appropriate to refrain from using a weight belt during weight training exercises in order to stimulate and strengthen these muscles for everyday activities.

Simply, weight belts tend to compensate for weak abdominal muscles. Before progressing to heavy loads, additional exercises to strengthen the abdominal muscles should be incorporated into the exercise program. These exercises will also allow the deep abdominal muscles to develop a pattern of muscle recruitment needed to generate a high IAP. The abdominal muscles, in particular, the rectus abdominus, can provide the body with its own natural lifting belt and, ultimately, decrease the potential for injury to the lower back.

Wrist Straps and Hooks

Grip fatigue is often a limiting factor when training the upper body with such exercises as lat pulldowns, upright rows, shrugs, bent-over rows and one-arm dumbbell rows. Straps and hooks can minimize grip strain, allowing the targeted muscle group to be worked more thoroughly. However, relying too heavily on the straps may result in injuries to the wrist and forearm.

Chalk

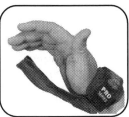

Chalk absorbs sweat and body oils that may be on weight lifting handles, bars and hands. It is used primarily to decrease the chance of hands slipping during heavy lifts. Chalk is not usually required as most machines have rubber handles.

.Basic Nutritional Considerations

The average person requires a variety of foods to provide the 50 nutrients essential to maintain everyday bodily functions. Optimal athletic performance relies heavily upon a sound understanding of basic nutritional requirements.

Energy Producing Nutrients

Food is composed of carbohydrates, proteins, fats, vitamins, and minerals. Carbohydrates, proteins, and fats are used in all processes that maintain body homeostasis. Vitamins and minerals aid in the conversion of nutrients to energy. Water is essential for temperature control, circulation, and urine production. Our daily food intake should be balanced in a way to provide all of these.

Carbohydrates

Carbohydrates are the most efficient source of fuel for the working muscles. They are utilized (or more correctly, burned) in the simplest form - glucose. Carbohydrates can be stored in limited amounts in the muscles and liver as glycogen. Excess carbohydrate is converted and stored as fat in the body. With regular aerobic training, the body may increase the stored amount of muscle glycogen and these stores are depleted at a slower rate during exercise.

Carbohydrates contribute 4 kcals of energy per gram. Carbohydrates should constitute about 55% of daily caloric intake. To calculate the number of grams of carbohydrates in a total daily intake of 2500 kcal:

- 55% of 2500 kcal (0.55 x 2500) = 1375 kcal
- 4 kcal / gram of carbohydrate (1375 / 4) = *344* grams

The two forms of carbohydrates are simple (sugars) and complex (fibre and starch). Complex carbohydrates (polysaccharides), often referred to as starches, are absorbed and digested by the body more slowly than simple carbohydrates. Simple carbohydrates include fructose (fruit sugar), sucrose (table sugar), and lactose (milk sugar) and several other sugars. Fruits are one of the richest natural sources of simple carbohydrates.

Good sources of complex carbohydrates are whole wheat pasta, kidney beans, lentils, apples, oranges, oats, and bran (e.g. Bran Flakes). Dietary intake high in complex carbohydrates is more nutrient dense (more nutrients than simple carbohydrates) and provide more B vitamins necessary for energy metabolism.

Dietary fibre, a complex carbohydrate, is divided into two categories - soluble and insoluble. Soluble fibre slows the transit time of the contents of the small intestine, allowing the nutrients to be absorbed more slowly. This can cause flatulence (gas) that subsides as the body becomes accustomed to the increased fibre intake. Soluble fibre is believed to help decrease blood cholesterol levels. Examples of soluble fibre include pectins and gums in foods such as fruits, vegetables, beans, peas, lentils, oatmeal, oat bran and corn bran. Insoluble fibre, or roughage, contributes to stool bulk by trapping water within its structure. It assists in shortening the transit time for the passage of food residues. The best source of insoluble fibre is wheat bran. Other sources include whole grains, corn kernels, fruit with edible seeds, cauliflower, broccoli, brussel sprouts, root vegetables, mushrooms and eggplants.

Fats

Fat is the highest concentrated source of energy equalling 9 kcal per gram. Dietary fat functions as an energy source, provides essential fatty acids (linoleic acid) and aids in the absorption and transport of fat-soluble vitamins (A,D,E and K). Factors that affect the degree of fat utilized during an exercise session are intensity, duration and exercise history (has the body been trained to utilize fat as a fuel effectively).

The recommended daily intake is 30% of total daily energy intake. To calculate the number of grams of fats in a total daily intake of 2500 kcal:

- 30% of 2500 kcal (0.30 x 2500) = 750 kcal
- 9 kcal / gram of fats (750 / 9) = **84** grams

Protein

Protein comprises approximately 45% of the tissue found in the human body. Proteins provide a structural role in the muscles, tendons and ligaments, skin, hair and nails, and are also used to maintain and repair these tissues. Protein is made of 20 amino acids of which 9 are essential (cannot be synthesized by the body) and 11 non-essential (can be synthesized by the body). Proteins play a role in athletic performance by assisting in oxygen transport to working muscles. A lesser role involves protein as an energy source during starvation or intense exercise. During intense aerobic sports, amino acids may supply up to 15% of the total energy used.

Protein requirements depend upon a person's size, gender, energy intake, degree of training, and intensity of training. The recommended daily intake of protein according to the Canada Food Guide is approximately 15%. To calculate the number of grams of proteins in a total daily intake of 2500 kcal:

- 15% of 2500 kcal (0.15 x 2500) = 375 kcal
- 4 kcal / gram of protein (375 / 4) = **94** grams

The effect of training on protein requirements is transient. Initially, protein loss increases with training, but the requirements return to normal after 5-14 days. Training may increase the efficiency of protein utilization.

Recent studies have found that the protein requirements of weight training athletes are actually similar to those of sedentary individuals due to the efficiency of protein utilization during weight training. Adequate protein stores and muscle growth can be obtained by 0.7-1.2g/kg/day of high quality dietary protein per day. Proteins have been classed as to their 'biological value' or quality. The biological value (BV) given to proteins describes how efficiently body tissue (e.g. muscle) can be made from food protein - the higher the value, the the more completely food protein is made into body protein. For example, whey isolate is considered to have the highest BV value (110-159), whole egg has a BV of 100, and peanuts have a BV of 55. Foods with a high BV contain all 9 essential amino acids. Low BV proteins are missing one or more of the essential amino acids or have disproportionate amounts of specific amino acids.

The Canada Food Guide and U.S. Food and Nutrition Board recommend between 0.7-0.8g/kg/day. However, research has found that some strength training athletes may require 1.2-2.0g/kg/day (or 12-15% of the total dietary intake). Ingesting more than 2g/kg/day is neither necessary nor beneficial. It is recommended that protein requirements be met primarily from dietary sources and not from supplementation.

Muscle tissue is comprised of about 20% protein. Studies have shown that strength and endurance athletes generally consume well in excess of the RDA (0.7g/kg/day for females and 0.8g/kg/day for males) for protein.

Protein digestion begins in the stomach where it is broken down by enzymes into amino acid chains called peptides. Most of the peptides are further broken down in the small intestine then absorbed into the bloodstream. They are then transported to the liver where they are used to synthesize serum proteins, transported to other organs for protein synthesis or used as a source of energy.

High protein diets may also be high in fat which may result in a slow or incomplete replacement of muscle glycogen and a diet high in protein may result in dehydration. So, drink lots of water.

Vitamins and Minerals

Vitamins are complex organic compounds existing in tiny quantities in food. They are essential for the optimal functioning of many physiological processes within the body. Vitamins and minerals play roles in enzymatic reactions including digestion and muscular contraction.

Although more research is needed to determine whether vitamins and minerals effect training, a regular dietary balance is necessary. A well-balanced diet will provide an adequate amount of vitamins and minerals.

B Complex Vitamins

This group of vitamins work together to aid in muscle contraction and relaxation, energy metabolism, healthy digestion and absorption of nutrients. They are water-soluble and, therefore, once tissues reach a saturation point, excess levels are excreted from the body. Studies have shown that large quantities are not beneficial, and vitamin supplementation has not proven to positively improve either aerobic or anaerobic potentials. They do not affect strength, speed or endurance.

Vitamin C

Vitamin C is involved in the synthesis of connective tissue, protein, and collagen. It is also involved in thyroxine synthesis (metabolism - controlling hormone), amino acid metabolism, iron absorption, and resistance to infection. Studies have shown that the enhancing effects of Vitamin C on athletic performance are contradictory. Some report that vitamin C may impair performance, yet other reports suggest that high doses are performance enhancing. Some examples of Vitamin C rich foods include citrus fruits, strawberries, broccoli, sweet peppers, brussels sprouts, cabbage, cauliflower, leafy greens, tomatoes, and potatoes. Overdoses of vitamin C may cause diarrhea and increase uric acid excretion.

Vitamins A, D, E, K

These vitamins are grouped together because they are all fat soluble vitamins. There are no specific storage depots in the body and any excess vitamins will be excreted when the body has received adequate amounts. These vitamins are stored in specific lipid-containing cells, usually located in the liver, and are taken when needed. At this time, there is no viable research between fat-soluble vitamins and athletic performance. Supplementation with these vitamins should only be advised by health professionals.

Calcium

The major functions of calcium include bone formation, bone strengthening, assisting nerve impulse transmission across cell membranes, muscle contraction, blood clotting, and the maintenance of tissue viability. Adequate calcium intake is especially important for children, young adults, and older women. While the intake of calcium in young adulthood is important, it is also important throughout life. As we age, there is an increased loss of calcium from our bones.

Iron

Iron is a component of hemoglobin and hemoglobin transports oxygen from the lungs to working muscles. An iron deficiency may result in poor oxygen supply to muscles which in turn reduces aerobic performance by decreasing energy production. Dietary consumption of iron has been found to be inadequate in some athletes because of inadequate intake, poor iron absorption, loss of iron via sweat, and gastrointestinal blood loss.

A condition referred to as sports-induced anemia appears often in athletes. It is associated with increased red blood cell destruction and decreased hemoglobin concentration at the beginning of a strenuous exercise program. Sports anaemia appears to be a transient condition that disappears when the body has adapted to the training regimen. Studies show that iron deficiency in athletes is more prevalent in female athletes than males because of regular menstrual losses. Other groups at risk of iron deficiency are vegetarian athletes, pubescent athletes (fast growth) and endurance athletes who experience a loss of iron through sweat and urine.

Only 10% of the iron in food is absorbed. The following are some recommendations for increasing dietary levels of iron:

- Eat lean cuts of red meat and dark poultry at least 3-4 times per week.
- Eat enriched or fortified breads, cereals, and pastas.
- Vitamin C enhances the absorption of iron.
- Avoid caffeinated tea and coffee because they inhibit iron absorption.

Water

Avoiding dehydration is the primary purpose of fluid intake. The general rule of thumb for water intake is 8 glasses per day, but is influenced by an individual's body surface area, environment, caloric intake, muscle mass and intensity and amount of exercise per day (sweating).

Proper hydration is important to counteract the fluid loss by the body. Water intake is also believed to help prevent the development of certain types of cancers (colon, bladder).

As a general hydration guideline, an individual should drink fluids prior, every 15 minutes during, and post exercise. A person should not wait for the thirst mechanism to indicates thirst because a person's body may already be in the early stages of dehydration. A person should also avoid caffeine beverages, supplements that contain high doses of caffeine, caffeine pills, salt pills, and alcohol or risk exercise dehydration.

Vegetarian Nutrition

There are several different types of vegetarian diets including:

- Those who eliminate red meat, but still include fish, poultry, eggs, and dairy products (lacto-ovo pecto-pollo vegetarian)
- Those who eliminate all meats, but still include eggs and dairy products (lacto-ovo vegetarian)
- Those who eliminate all meats, eggs, and dairy products (vegan vegetarian).

Most vegetarian diets will meet the requirements for carbohydrates, however, meeting adequate protein requirements is more of a concern. Vegetarian diets that include some animal products will supply a small amount of high quality protein, but vegan vegetarian diets must chose protein products wisely in order to intake the best plant protein available. Other nutrient concerns of vegetarian diets include the possibility of injesting inadequate quantities of vitamin B12, iron, zinc, and calcium. Vitamin B12 can be obtained by eating milk, cheese, eggs, and fortified soy products or brewer's yeast. Iron may be enhanced by choosing iron-rich foods and consuming them with foods containing vitamin C.

Stretching

Full Body

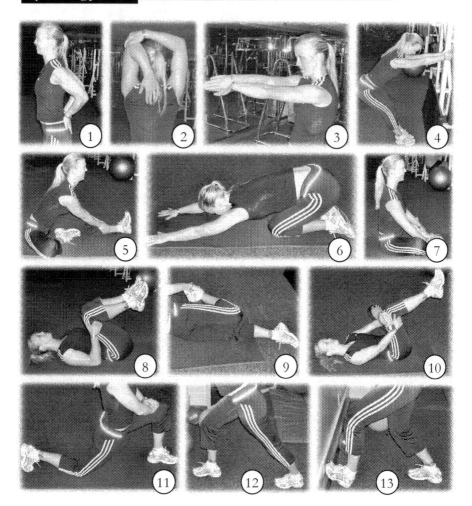

Here are 13 basic stretches to perform pre and/or post workout:
1. Pectorals Stretch
2. Triceps Stretch
3. Mid Back Stretch #1
4. Mid Back Stretch #2
5. Hamstrings & Lower Back Stretch
6. Lower/Mid Back & Shoulder Stretch
7. Adductors Stretch
8. Glutes & Lower Back Stretch
9. Quads & Hip Flexors Stretch
10. Glutes, Piriformis & Lower Back Stretch
11. Hip Flexor Stretch
12. Gastrocnemius Stretch
13. Soleus Stretch

Exercises

Chest

Bench Press (Barbell, Flat) - compound, free weights
Pectoralis, Triceps, Anterior Deltoids
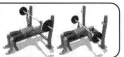

Bench Press (Barbell, Decline) - compound, free weights
Pectoralis, Triceps, Anterior Deltoids
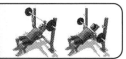

Bench Press (Barbell, Incline) - compound, free weights
Pectoralis, Triceps, Anterior Deltoids
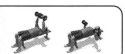

Bench Press (Dumbbell, Flat) - compound, free weights
Pectoralis, Triceps, Anterior Deltoids
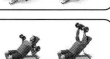

Bench Press (DB, Decline) - compound, free weights
Pectoralis, Triceps, Anterior Deltoids
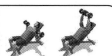

Bench Press (DB, Incline) - compound, free weights
Pectoralis, Triceps, Anterior Deltoids
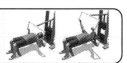

Bench Press (Machine, Flat) - compound, machine
Pectoralis, Triceps, Anterior Deltoids
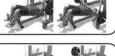

Bench Press (Smith Machine, Flat) - compound, machine
Pectoralis, Triceps, Anterior Deltoids
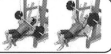

Bench Press (Smith Mach, Decline) - compound, machine
Pectoralis, Triceps, Anterior Deltoids
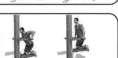

Bench Press (Smith Machine, Incline) –compound, machine
Pectoralis, Triceps, Anterior Deltoids

Chest Dips (Machine) - compound, machine
Pectoralis, Triceps, Anterior Deltoids

Chest Dips (Parallel Bars) - compound, no weight
Pectoralis major, Triceps, Anterior Deltoids

Flyes (Cable, Bent Over) - isolation, pulleys
Pectoralis major, Anterior Deltoids, *Triceps, Forearms, Biceps*

Flyes (Cable, Decline) - isolation, pulleys
Pectoralis major, Anterior Deltoids, *Triceps, Forearms*

Flyes (Cable, Flat Bench) - isolation, pulleys
Pectoralis major, Anterior Deltoids, *Triceps, Forearms, Biceps*

Flyes (Cable, Incline) - isolation, pulleys
Pectoralis major, Anterior Deltoids, *Triceps, Forearms, Biceps*

Flyes (Cable, Upright) - isolation, pulleys
Pectoralis major, Anterior Deltoids, *Triceps, Forearms, Biceps*

Flyes (Dumbbell, Decline) - isolation, free weights
Pectoralis major, Anterior Deltoids, *Triceps, Forearms, Biceps*

Flyes (Dumbbell, Flat Bench) - isolation, free weights
Pectoralis major, Anterior Deltoids, *Triceps, Forearms, Biceps*

Flyes (Dumbbell, Incline) - isolation, free weights
Pectoralis major, Anterior Deltoids, *Triceps, Forearms, Biceps*

Flyes (Machine, Seated) - isolation, machine
Pectoralis major, Anterior Deltoids, *Biceps*

Machine Chest Press (Decline) - compound, machine
Pectoralis, Triceps, Anterior Deltoids

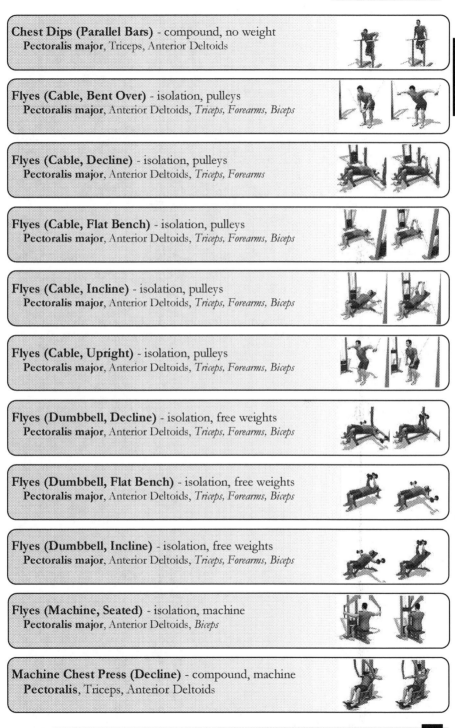

Machine Chest Press (Incline) - compound, machine
   Pectoralis major, Triceps, Anterior Deltoids

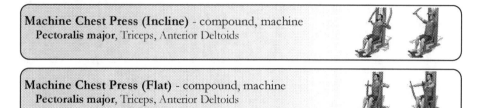

Machine Chest Press (Flat) - compound, machine
   Pectoralis major, Triceps, Anterior Deltoids

Arm Curls (Cable, One Arm) - isolation, pulleys
   Pectoralis major, Anterior Deltoids

Push-Ups - compound, no weight
   Pectoralis major, Triceps, Anterior Deltoids, *abdominals*

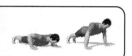

Exercises Back / Lats

Bent Over Row (Barbell) - compound, free weights
Lats, Traps, Post Delt, Bi's, *Erector spinae, Hamstrings, Glute max*

Bent Over Row (DB, One-Arm) - compound, free weights
Latissimus dorsi, Trapezius, Posterior Deltoids, Biceps

Bent Over Row (Smith Machine) - compound, machine
Lats, Traps, Post Delt, Bi's, *Erector spinae, Hamstrings, Glute max*

Chin-ups (Front, Close Grip) - compound, no weight
Latissimus dorsi, Trapezius, Posterior Deltoids, Biceps

Chin-ups (Front, Underhand) - compound, no weight
Latissimus dorsi, Trapezius, Posterior Deltoids, Biceps

Chin-ups (Front, Wide-Grip) - compound, no weight
Lat. dorsi, Forearm muscles, Trapezius, Post Deltoids, Biceps

Chin-ups (Machine Assisted) - compound, machine
Lat. dorsi, Forearm muscles, Trapezius, Post Deltoids, Biceps

Chin-ups (Rear, Wide Grip) - compound, no weight
Latissimus dorsi, Trapezius, Pectoralis, Biceps

Cross-Bench Pullovers (Barbell) - isolation, free weights
Latissimus dorsi, Triceps, Pectoralis, Posterior Deltoids

Cross-Bench Pullovers (DB) - isolation, free weights
Latissimus dorsi, **Pectoralis**, Triceps, Posterior Deltoids

Lying Row (Dumbbell, 2-Arm) - compound, free weights
Latissimus dorsi, Trapezius, Posterior Deltoids, Biceps

Machine Pullovers - isolation, machine
Latissimus dorsi, Triceps, Pectoralis, Post. Deltoids, *Trapezius*

Pulldowns (Front, Close-Grip) - compound, pulleys
Latissimus dorsi, Forearm, Trapezius, Post. Deltoids, Biceps

Pulldowns (Front, Underhand) - compound, pulleys
Latissimus dorsi, Forearm, Trapezius, Post. Deltoids, Biceps

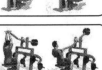

Pulldowns (Front, Wide-Grip) - compound, pulleys
Latissimus dorsi, Forearm, Trapezius, Post. Deltoids, Biceps

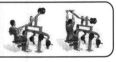

Pulldowns (Machine, Close Grip) - compound, machine
Latissimus dorsi, Forearm, Trapezius, Post. Deltoids, Biceps

Pulldowns (Machine, Wide Grip) - compound, machine
Latissimus dorsi, Forearm, Trapezius, Post. Deltoids, Biceps

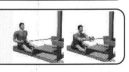

Pulldowns (Rear) - compound, pulleys
Latissimus dorsi, Forearm muscles, Trapezius, Biceps

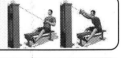

Seated Row (Cable, Low) - compound, pulleys
Latissimus dorsi, Trapezius, Erector spinae, Posterior Deltoids,
Biceps, *Hamstrings, Gluteus maximus*

Seated Row (Cable, High) - compound, pulleys
Latissimus dorsi, Trapezius, Erector spinae, Posterior Deltoids,
Biceps, *Hamstrings, Gluteus maximus*

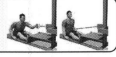

Seated Row (Cable, One Arm) - compound, pulleys
Latissimus dorsi, Trapezius, Erector spinae, Posterior Deltoids,
Biceps, *Hamstrings, Gluteus maximus*

Seated Row (Cable, Wide Grip) - compound, pulleys
Latissimus dorsi, Trapezius, Erector spinae, Posterior Deltoids,
Biceps, *Hamstrings, Gluteus maximus*

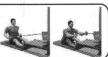

Row (Machine) - compound, machine
Latissimus dorsi, Trapezius, Posterior Deltoids, Biceps
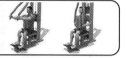

Row (Machine, High) - compound, machine
Latissimus dorsi, Trapezius, Posterior Deltoids, Biceps
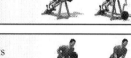

Bent-over Row (Machine, Incline) - compound, machine
Latissimus dorsi, Trapezius, Posterior Deltoids, Biceps
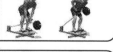

T-Bar Row (Barbell, V-Grip) - compound, free weights
Latissimus dorsi, Trapezius, Posterior Deltoids, Biceps, *Erector spinae, Hamstrings, Gluteus maximus*

T-Bar Row (Machine, Close Grip) - compound, machine
Latissimus dorsi, Trapezius, Posterior Deltoids, Biceps, *Erector spinae, Hamstrings, Gluteus maximus*

T-Bar Row (Machine, Wide Grip) - compound, machine
Latissimus dorsi, Trapezius, Posterior Deltoids, Biceps, *Erector spinae, Hamstrings, Gluteus maximus*
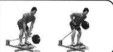

Exercises Lower Back

Deadlifts - compound, free weights
Erector spinae, Gluteus maximus, Quadriceps, Hip
Adductors, Calves

Deadlifts (Smith Machine) - compound, machine
Erector spinae, Gluteus maximus, Quadriceps, Hip
Adductors, Calves

Back Extensions (45 degree) - isolation, no weight
Erector spinae, Hamstrings, Gluteus maximus, Hip
Adductors

Machine Low Back Extensions - isolation, machine
Erector spinae, *Quadriceps, Gluteus maximus*

Stiff Leg Deadlifts - compound, free weights
Erector spinae, Gluteus maximus, Hamstrings, Adductors,
Quadriceps

Straight Leg Deadlifts - compound, free weights
Erector spinae, Hamstrings, Gluteus maximus, Adductors

Straight Leg Deadlifts (DB) - compound, free weights
Erector spinae, Hamstrings, Gluteus maximus, Adductors

Exercises

Biceps

Arm Curls (Barbell) - isolation, free weights
Biceps, Brachialis, *Forearm muscles, Trapezius, Anterior Deltoids*

Arm Curls (Cable) - isolation, pulleys
Biceps, Brachialis, *Forearm muscles, Trapezius, Anterior Deltoids*

Arm Curls (Cable, One Arm) - isolation, pulleys
Biceps, Brachialis, *Forearm muscles, Trapezius, Anterior Deltoids*

Arm Curls (Dumbbell, Incline) - isolation, free weights
Biceps, Brachialis, Forearm muscles, *Anterior Deltoids*

Arm Curls (Dumbbell, Seated) - isolation, free weights
Biceps, Brachialis, *Forearm muscles, Trapezius, Anterior Deltoids*

Arm Curls (Dumbbell, Standing) - isolation, free weights
Biceps, Brachialis, *Forearm muscles, Trapezius, Anterior Deltoids*

Arm Curls (Machine) - isolation, machine
Biceps, Brachialis, *Forearm muscles, Anterior Deltoids*

Concentration Curls - isolation, free weights
Brachialis, Biceps, *Forearm muscles, Trapezius*

Preacher Curls (Barbell) - isolation, free weights
Brachialis, Biceps, *Forearm muscles*

Preacher Curls (Cable) - isolation, pulleys
Brachialis, Biceps, *Forearm muscles*

Preacher Curls (Dumbbell) - isolation, free weights
Brachialis, Biceps, *Forearm muscles*

Exercises

Triceps

Bench Dips - compound, no weight
Triceps, Latissimus dorsi, Anterior Deltoids, Pectoralis, *Arms, Trapezius*

Cable Pushdowns - isolation, pulleys
Triceps, *Forearm muscles, Latissimus dorsi, Shoulders, Pectoralis*

Cable Pushdowns (Heavy) - isolation, pulleys
Triceps, *Forearm muscles, Latissimus dorsi, Trapezius, Shoulders*

Cable Pushdowns (One Arm) - isolation, pulleys
Triceps, *Latissimus dorsi, Shoulders, Pectoralis*

Cable Pushdowns (Rope) - isolation, pulleys
Triceps, *Forearm, Latissimus dorsi, Traps, Pectoralis, Post Deltoids*

Close-Grip Bench (BB) - compound, free weights
Triceps, Anterior Deltoids, Pectoralis

Close-Grip Bench (BB, Incline) - compound, free weights
Triceps, Anterior Deltoids, Pectoralis

Close-Grip Bench (Smith) - compound, machine
Triceps, *Anterior Deltoids, Pectoralis*

Push-Ups (Narrow Hands) - compound, no weight
Triceps, Pectoralis, Rectus abdominis, Quadriceps

Seated Narrow Grip Press - compound, machine
Triceps, Anterior Deltoids, Pectoralis

Triceps Dips (Assisted) - compound, machine
Triceps, Latissimus dorsi, Anterior Deltoids, Pectoralis

Triceps Dips (Machine) - compound, machine
Triceps, Latissimus dorsi, Anterior Deltoids, Pectoralis

Triceps Dips (Parallel Bars) - compound, no weight
Triceps, Lat. dorsi, Anterior Deltoids, Pectoralis, Trapezius

Triceps Extensions (Barbell) - isolation, free weights
Triceps, Forearm muscles, Anterior Deltoids, Pectoralis

Triceps Extensions (BB, Lying) - isolation, free weights
Triceps, Forearm muscles, Latissimus dorsi, Shoulders, Pectoralis

Triceps Extensions (Cable) - isolation, pulleys
Triceps, Forearm muscles, Anterior Deltoids, Pectoralis

Triceps Extensions (Cable, Bent-over) - isolation, pulleys
Triceps, Forearm muscles, Anterior Deltoids, Pectoralis

Triceps Extensions (Cable, Incline) - isolation, pulleys
Triceps, Forearm muscles, Latissimus dorsi, Anterior Deltoids, Pectoralis

Triceps Extensions (Cable, Kneeling) - isolation, pulleys
Triceps, Forearm muscles

Triceps Extensions (Cable, Lying) - isolation, pulleys
Triceps, Forearm muscles, Latissimus dorsi, Shoulders, Pectoralis

Triceps Extensions (Dumbbell) - isolation, free weights
Triceps, Forearm muscles, Anterior Deltoids, Pectoralis

Triceps Extensions (DB, Incline) - isolation, free weights
Triceps, Latissimus dorsi, Shoulders, Pectoralis

Triceps Extensions (DB, Lying) - isolation, free weights
Triceps, *Latissimus dorsi, Shoulders, Pectoralis*

Triceps Extensions (DB, 1-Arm) - isolation, free weights
Triceps, *Forearm muscles*

Triceps Extensions (Machine) - isolation, machine
Triceps, *Pectoralis, Posterior Deltoids*

Triceps Kickbacks (Dumbbell) - isolation, free weights
Triceps, *Latissimus dorsi, Trapezius, Posterior Deltoids*

Underhand Press (Barbell) - compound, free weights
Triceps, Anterior Deltoids, Pectoralis, *Forearm muscles*

Exercises

Shoulder

Anterior Deltoid

Arnold Press - compound, free weights
Anterior Deltoid, Triceps, Trapezius, Medial Deltoid

Behind Neck Press (Barbell) - compound, free weights
Anterior Deltoid, Triceps, Trapezius, Medial Deltoid

Behind Neck Press (Smith Machine) - compound, machine
Anterior Deltoid, Triceps, Trapezius, Medial Deltoid

Front Raises (Barbell) - isolation, free weights
Anterior Deltoid, Trapezius, Pectoralis, Medial Deltoid

Front Raises (Cable) - isolation, pulleys
Anterior Deltoid, Trapezius, Pectoralis, Medial Deltoid

Front Raises (Dumbbell) - isolation, free weights
Anterior Deltoid, Trapezius, Pectoralis, Medial Deltoid

Shoulder Press (Barbell) - compound, free weights
Anterior Deltoid, Triceps, Trapezius, Pectoralis, Medial Deltoid

Shoulder Press (DB, Seated) - compound, free weights
Anterior Deltoid, Triceps, Trapezius, Pectoralis, Medial Deltoid

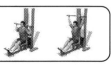

Shoulder Press (Machine) - compound, machine
Anterior Deltoid, Triceps, Trapezius, Pectoralis, Medial Deltoid

Medial Deltoid

Lateral Raises (Cable) - isolation, pulleys
Lateral Deltoid, Trapezius, Anterior Deltoids

Lateral Raises (Dumbbell) - isolation, free weights
Lateral Deltoid, Trapezius, Anterior Deltoids

Lateral Raises (Machine) - isolation, machine
Lateral Deltoid, Trapezius, Anterior Deltoids

Upright Rows (Barbell) - compound, free weights
Lateral Deltoid, Trapezius (upper), Anterior Deltoids, Biceps

Upright Rows (Cable) - compound, pulleys
Lateral Deltoid, Trapezius (upper), Anterior Deltoids, Biceps

Upright Rows (Dumbbell) - compound, free weights
Lateral Deltoid, Trapezius (upper), Anterior Deltoids, Biceps

Posterior Deltoid

Bent Over Raises (Cable) - isolation, pulleys
Posterior Deltoids, Trapezius, Rhomboids, Medial Deltoid

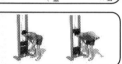

Bent Over Raises (Cable, One Arm) - isolation, pulleys
Posterior Deltoids, Trapezius, Rhomboids, Medial Deltoid

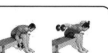

Bent Over Raises (DB, Standing) - isolation, free weights
Posterior Deltoids, Trapezius, Rhomboids, Medial Deltoid

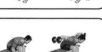

Bent Over Raises (DB, Seated) - isolation, free weights
Posterior Deltoids, Trapezius, Rhomboids, Medial Deltoid

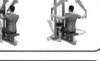

Machine Seated Rear Raises - isolation, machine
Posterior Deltoids, Trapezius, Rhomboids, Medial Deltoid

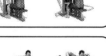

Rear Delt Row (Barbell) - compound, free weights
Posterior Deltoids, Trapezius, Rhomboids, Medial Deltoid,
biceps

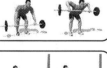

Rear Delt Row (Cable) - compound, pulleys
Posterior Deltoids, Trapezius, Rhomboids, Medial Deltoid,
biceps

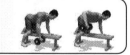

Rear Delt Row (Dumbbell) - compound, free weights
Posterior Deltoids, Trapezius, Rhomboids, Medial Deltoid,
biceps

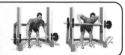

Rear Delt Row (Smith Machine) - compound, machine
Posterior Deltoids, Trapezius, Rhomboids, Medial Deltoid,
biceps

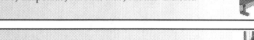

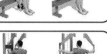

Exercises Upper Traps

Shrugs (Barbell) - isolation, free weights
  Trapezius (superior & middle), *Levator scapulae*

Shrugs (Low Cable) - isolation, pulleys
  Trapezius (superior & middle), *Levator scapulae*

Shrugs (Dumbbell) - isolation, free weights
  Trapezius (superior & middle), *Levator scapulae*

Shrugs (Machine) - isolation, machine
  Trapezius (superior & middle), *Levator scapulae*

Shrugs (Smith Machine) - isolation, machine
  Trapezius (superior & middle), *Levator scapulae*

Exercises

Forearm

Hammer Curls (Cable, Rope) - isolation, pulleys
Forearm muscles, Brachialis, Biceps

Hammer Curls (Dumbbell) - isolation, free weights
Forearm muscles, Brachialis, Biceps

Reverse Arm Curls (Barbell) - isolation, free weights
Forearm muscles, Brachialis, Biceps

Reverse Arm Curls (Cable) - isolation, pulleys
Forearm muscles, Brachialis, Biceps

Reverse Arm Curls (DB, Standing) - isolation, free weights
Forearm muscles, Brachialis, Biceps

Reverse Preacher Curls (Barbell) - isolation, free weights
Forearm muscles, Brachialis, Biceps

Reverse Preacher Curls (Cable) - isolation, pulleys
Forearm muscles, Brachialis, Biceps

Prontated Wrist Curls (Barbell) - isolation, free weights
Forearm muscles (extensors)

Supinated Wrist Curls (Barbell) - isolation, free weights
Forearm muscles (flexors)

Prontated Wrist Curls (DB) - isolation, free weights
Forearm muscles (extensors)

Supinated Wrist Curls (DB) - isolation, free weights
Forearm muscles (flexors)

Exercises Abdominals

Bicycle Crunches - isolation, no weight
  Rectus abdominis, Obliques

Cable Crunches (Kneeling) - isolation, pulleys
  Rectus abdominis, Obliques

Crunches - isolation, no weight
  Rectus abdominis, Obliques

Crunches With Legs - isolation, no weight
  Rectus abdominis, Obliques, Hip Flexors

Hooked Feet Curl Ups - compound, no weight
  Rectus abdominis, Obliques, Hip flexors

Leg Raises (Flat Bench) - isolation, no weight
  Rectus abdominis, Hip Flexors, Obliques

Leg Raises (Hanging) - isolation, no weight
  Rectus abdominis, Hip Flexors, Obliques

Leg Raises (Incline Bench) - isolation, no weight
  Rectus abdominis, Hip Flexors, Obliques

Leg Raises (Roman Chair) - isolation, no weight
  Rectus abdominis, Hip Flexors, Obliques, Latissimus dorsi,
  Trapezius, Pectoralis

Leg-Hip Raises (Hanging) - compound, no weight
  Rectus abdominis, Hip Flexors, Obliques

Leg-Hip Raises (Hanging, Straight Legs) - isolation
  Rectus abdominis, Hip Flexors, Obliques

Leg-Hip Raises (Incline) - compound, no weight
Rectus abdominis, Obliques, Hip flexors

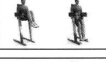

Leg-Hip Raises (Parallel Bar) - compound, no weight
Rectus abdominis, Obliques, Hip flexors

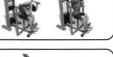

Machine Crunches - isolation, machine
Rectus abdominis, Obliques

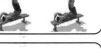

Reverse Crunches - isolation, no weight
Rectus abdominis, *Obliques*, Hip flexors

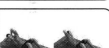

Side Twist (Lying) - isolation, no weight
Rectus abdominis, Obliques, Hip flexors

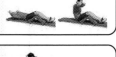

Hooked Feet Sit-Ups - compound, no weight
Rectus abdominis, Obliques, Hip flexors

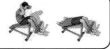

Sit-Ups (Incline Bench) - compound, no weight
Rectus abdominis, Obliques, Hip flexors

Twisting Crunches - isolation, no weight
Rectus abdominis, Obliques

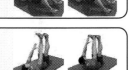

Vertical Leg Crunches - isolation, no weight
Rectus abdominis, Obliques, Hip flexors

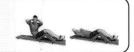

Twisting Hooked Feet Sit-Up - compound, no weight
Rectus abdominis, Obliques, Hip flexors

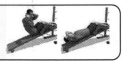

Twisting Sit-Up (Incline Bench) - compound, no weight
Rectus abdominis, Obliques, Hip flexors

45° Side Bends - isolation, no weight
Obliques, Quadratus lumborum, Erector spinae

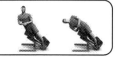

Bicycle Crunches - isolation, no weight
Rectus abdominis, Obliques

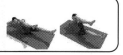

Rotation Machine - isolation, machine
Obliques, Quadratus lumborum, Erector spinae

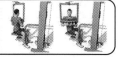

Russian Twists - isolation, no weight
Obliques, Rectus abdominis, Quadratus lumborum, Erector spinae

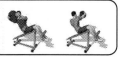

Side Bends (Cable) - isolation, pulleys
Obliques, Rectus abdominis, Quadratus lumborum, Erector spinae

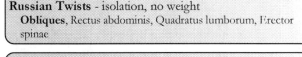

Side Bends (Dumbbell) - isolation, free weights
Obliques, Rectus abdominis, Quadratus lumborum, Erector spinae

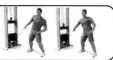

Side Lying Crunches - isolation, no weight
Obliques, Rectus abdominis, Quadratus lumborum, Erector spinae

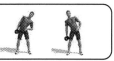

Side Twists (Lying) - isolation, no weight
Rectus abdominis, Obliques

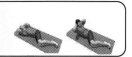

Side Twist Crunches (Lying) - isolation, no weight
Rectus abdominis, Obliques

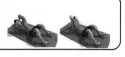

Twisting Crunches (Incline Bench) - isolation, no weight
Rectus abdominis, Obliques, Hip flexors

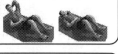

Twisting Sit-Up (Incline Bench) - compound, no weight
Rectus abdominis, Obliques, Hip flexors

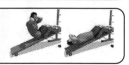

Exercises

Quads

Hack Squats (Machine) - compound, machine
Quadriceps, Gluteus maximus, Hip Adductors, Tibialis anterior
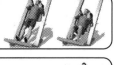

Front Squats - compound, free weights
Quadriceps, Gluteus maximus, Hip Adductors, Calves, *Trapezius, Erector spinae*
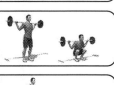

Front Squats (Smith Machine) - compound, machine
Quadriceps, Gluteus maximus, Hip Adductors, Calves, *Trapezius, Erector spinae*
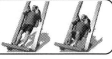

Full Squats - compound, free weights
Quadriceps, Gluteus maximus, Hip Adductors, Calves, *Trapezius, Erector spinae*
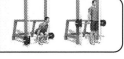

Hack Squats (Barbell) - compound, free weights
Quadriceps, Gluteus maximus, Hip Adductors, Calves, *Trapezius, Erector spinae*
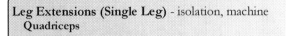

Hack Squats (Machine) - compound, machine
Quadriceps, Gluteus maximus, Hip Adductors, Calves
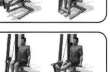

Hack Squats (Smith Machine) - compound, machine
Quadriceps, Gluteus maximus, Hip Adductors, Calves, *Trapezius, Erector spinae*
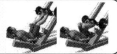

Leg Extensions - isolation, machine
Quadriceps
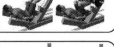

Leg Extensions (Single Leg) - isolation, machine
Quadriceps

Incline Leg Press - compound, machine
Quadriceps, Gluteus maximus, Hip Adductors, Calves
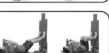

Leg Press (Lying) - compound, machine
Quadriceps, Gluteus maximus, Hip Adductors, Calves
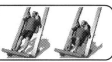

Leg Press (Seated) - compound, machine
Quadriceps, Gluteus maximus, Hip Adductors, Calves, *hamstrings*

Lunges (Dumbbell) - compound, no weight
Quadriceps, Gluteus maximus, Hip Adductors, Calves, *Erector spinae, hamstrings*

Lunges (Barbell) - compound, free weights
Quadriceps, Gluteus maximus, Hip Adductors, Calves, *hamstrings*

Lunges (Smith Machine) - compound, machine
Quadriceps, Gluteus maximus, Hip Adductors, Calves, *Erector spinae, hamstrings*

Stepback Lunges (Barbell) - compound, free weights
Quadriceps, Gluteus maximus, Hip Adductors, Calves, *Erector spinae, hamstrings*

Stepback Lunges (Dumbbell) - compound, free weights
Quadriceps, Gluteus maximus, Hip Adductors, Calves, *Erector spinae, hamstrings*

Sissy Squats - isolation, free weights
Quadriceps, *Rectus abdominis, Gluteus maximus, Calves*

Squats - compound, free weights
Quadriceps, Gluteus maximus, Hip Adductors, Calves, *Erector spinae*

Squats (Dumbbells) - compound, free weights
Quadriceps, Gluteus maximus, Hip Adductors, Calves, *Erector spinae*

Squats (Machine) - compound, machine
Quadriceps, Gluteus maximus, Hip Adductors, Calves, *Erector spinae*

Sumo Squats (Single DB) - compound, free weights
Quadriceps, Gluteus maximus, Hip Adductors, Calves, *Erector spinae*

Squats (Smith Machine) - compound, machine
Quadriceps, Gluteus maximus, Hip Adductors, Calves, *Erector spinae*

Step-up (Barbell) - compound, free weights
Quadriceps, Gluteus maximus, Hip Adductors, Calves, *Erector spinae*

Step-up (Dumbbell) - compound, free weights
Quadriceps, Gluteus maximus, Hip Adductors, Calves, *Erector spinae*

Exercises Hamstrings

Glute-Ham Raise (Plate) - isolation, free weights
Hamstrings, Hip Adductors, Gluteus maximus, Gastrocnemius, *Erector spinae*

Hamstring Raises (Plate) - isolation, free weights
Hamstrings, Hip Adductors, Gastrocnemius, *Erector spinae*, *Gluteus maximus*

Back Extensions (45 degree) - isolation, no weight
Erector spinae, Hamstrings, Gluteus maximus, Hip Adductors

Kneeling Leg Curls - isolation, machine
Hamstrings, Hip Adductors, Calves, *Gluteus maximus*

Lying Leg Curls - isolation, machine
Hamstrings, Hip Adductors, Gastrocnemius

Seated Leg Curls - isolation, machine
Hamstrings, Hip Adductors, Gastrocnemius

Standing Leg Curls - isolation, machine
Hamstrings, Hip Adductors, Calves, *Gluteus maximus*

Straight Leg Deadlifts - compound, free weights
Erector spinae, Hamstrings, Gluteus maximus, Hip Adductors

Straight Leg Deadlifts (DB) - compound, free weights
Erector spinae, Hamstrings, Gluteus maximus, Hip Adductors

Straight Leg & Back Deadlifts - compound, free weights
Hamstrings, Gluteus maximus, Erector spinae, Hip Adductors

Straight Leg & Back Deadlifts - compound, free weights
Hamstrings, Gluteus maximus, Erector spinae, Hip Adductors

Exercises

Calves

Gastrocnemius

Incline Calf Presses - isolation, machine
Gastrocnemius, Soleus

Lying Calf Press - isolation, machine
Gastrocnemius, Soleus

Standing Calf Raises (Smith/BB) - isolation, free weights
Gastrocnemius, Soleus

Standing Calf Raises (Dumbbell) - isolation, free weights
Gastrocnemius, Soleus

Standing Calf Raises (Machine) - isolation, machine
Gastrocnemius, Soleus

Soleus

Seated Calf Raises (Barbell) - isolation, free weights
Soleus, Gastrocnemius

Seated Calf Raises (Dumbbell) - isolation, free weights
Soleus, Gastrocnemius

Seated Calf Raises (Machine) - isolation, machine
Soleus, Gastrocnemius

Seated Calf Raises (Plate) - isolation, free weights
Soleus, Gastrocnemius

Exercises

Abductors
Adductors

Hip Abductors

Hip Abductions (Low Cable) - isolation, pulleys
Hip Abductors
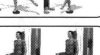

Hip Abductions (Machine, Seated) - isolation, machine
Hip Abductors
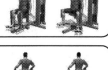

Hip Abductions (Machine, Standing) - isolation, machine
Hip Abductors

Hip Adductors

Hip Adductions (Cable) - isolation, pulleys
Hip Adductors
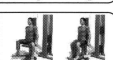

Hip Adductions (Machine, Seated) - isolation, machine
Hip Adductors

Hip Adductions (Machine, Standing) - isolation, machine
Hip Adductors

My Workout Log

How to fill out the Journal:

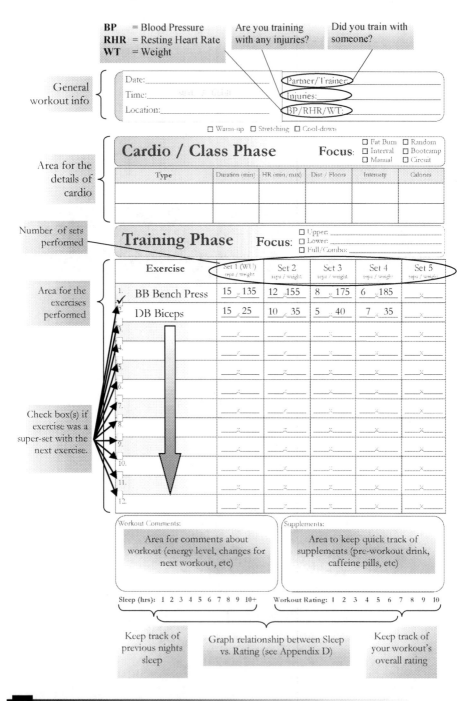

BP = Blood Pressure
RHR = Resting Heart Rate
WT = Weight

Are you training with any injuries?

Did you train with someone?

General workout info

Date:_____
Time:_____
Location:_____

Partner/Trainer:_____
Injuries:_____
BP/RHR/WT:_____

☐ Warm-up ☐ Stretching ☐ Cool-down

Area for the details of cardio

Cardio / Class Phase

Focus:
☐ Fat Burn ☐ Random
☐ Interval ☐ Bootcamp
☐ Manual ☐ Circuit

Type	Duration (min)	HR (min/max)	Dist / Floors	Intensity	Calories

Number of sets performed

Training Phase

Focus:
☐ Upper:_____
☐ Lower:_____
☐ Full/Combo:_____

Area for the exercises performed

Check box(s) if exercise was a super-set with the next exercise.

Exercise	Set 1 (WU) reps / weight	Set 2 reps / weight	Set 3 reps / weight	Set 4 reps / weight	Set 5 reps / weight
1. BB Bench Press	15 / 135	12 / 155	8 / 175	6 / 185	__ x __
2. DB Biceps	15 / 25	10 / 35	5 / 40	7 / 35	__ x __
3.	/	/	/	x	x
4.	/	/	/	x	x
5.	/	/	/	x	x
6.	/	/	/	x	x
7.	/	/	/	x	x
8.	/	/	/	x	x
9.	/	/	/	x	x
10.	/	/	/	x	x
11.	/	/	/	x	x
12.	/	/	/	x	x

Workout Comments:
Area for comments about workout (energy level, changes for next workout, etc)

Supplements:
Area to keep quick track of supplements (pre-workout drink, caffeine pills, etc)

Sleep (hrs): 1 2 3 4 5 6 7 8 9 10+

Workout Rating: 1 2 3 4 5 6 7 8 9 10

Keep track of previous nights sleep

Graph relationship between Sleep vs. Rating (see Appendix D)

Keep track of your workout's overall rating

Partner/Trainer:_____   Date:_____

Injuries:_____   Time:_____ start / finish

BP/RHR/WT:_____   Location:_____

☐ Warm-up   ☐ Stretching   ☐ Cool-down

Cardio / Class Phase   Focus:

☐ Fat Burn   ☐ Random
☐ Interval   ☐ Bootcamp
☐ Manual   ☐ Circuit

Type	Duration (min)	HR (min/max)	Dist / Floors	Intensity	Calories

Training Phase   Focus:

☐ Upper: _____
☐ Lower: _____
☐ Full/Combo: _____

Exercise	Set 1 (WU) reps / weight	Set 2 reps / weight	Set 3 reps / weight	Set 4 reps / weight	Set 5 reps / weight
1.	___X___	___X___	___X___	___X___	___X___
2.	___X___	___X___	___X___	___X___	___X___
3.	___X___	___X___	___X___	___X___	___X___
4.	___X___	___X___	___X___	___X___	___X___
5.	___X___	___X___	___X___	___X___	___X___
6.	___X___	___X___	___X___	___X___	___X___
7.	___X___	___X___	___X___	___X___	___X___
8.	___X___	___X___	___X___	___X___	___X___
9.	___X___	___X___	___X___	___X___	___X___
10.	___X___	___X___	___X___	___X___	___X___
11.	___X___	___X___	___X___	___X___	___X___
12.	___X___	___X___	___X___	___X___	___X___

Workout Comments:

Supplements:

Sleep (hrs): 1 2 3 4 5 6 7 8 9 10+   Workout Rating: 1 2 3 4 5 6 7 8 9 10

Date:_____   Partner/Trainer:_____

Time:_____ start / finish   Injuries:_____

Location:_____ BP/RHR/WT:_____

☐ Warm-up   ☐ Stretching   ☐ Cool-down

Cardio / Class Phase   Focus:

☐ Fat Burn   ☐ Random
☐ Interval   ☐ Bootcamp
☐ Manual   ☐ Circuit

Type	Duration (min)	HR (min/max)	Dist / Floors	Intensity	Calories

Training Phase   Focus:

☐ Upper: _____
☐ Lower: _____
☐ Full/Combo: _____

Exercise	Set 1 (WU) reps / weight	Set 2 reps / weight	Set 3 reps / weight	Set 4 reps / weight	Set 5 reps / weight
1. ☐	___X___	___X___	___X___	___X___	___X___
2. ☐	___X___	___X___	___X___	___X___	___X___
3. ☐	___X___	___X___	___X___	___X___	___X___
4. ☐	___X___	___X___	___X___	___X___	___X___
5. ☐	___X___	___X___	___X___	___X___	___X___
6. ☐	___X___	___X___	___X___	___X___	___X___
7. ☐	___X___	___X___	___X___	___X___	___X___
8. ☐	___X___	___X___	___X___	___X___	___X___
9. ☐	___X___	___X___	___X___	___X___	___X___
10. ☐	___X___	___X___	___X___	___X___	___X___
11. ☐	___X___	___X___	___X___	___X___	___X___
12.	___X___	___X___	___X___	___X___	___X___

Workout Comments:

Supplements:

Sleep (hrs): 1 2 3 4 5 6 7 8 9 10+   Workout Rating: 1 2 3 4 5 6 7 8 9 10

Partner/Trainer:_____

Injuries:_____

BP/RHR/WT:_____

Date:_____

Time:_____ start / finish

Location:_____

☐ Warm-up   ☐ Stretching   ☐ Cool-down

Cardio / Class Phase   Focus:

☐ Fat Burn   ☐ Random
☐ Interval   ☐ Bootcamp
☐ Manual   ☐ Circuit

Type	Duration (min)	HR (min/max)	Dist / Floors	Intensity	Calories

Training Phase   Focus:

☐ Upper: _____
☐ Lower: _____
☐ Full/Combo: _____

Exercise	Set 1 (WU) reps / weight	Set 2 reps / weight	Set 3 reps / weight	Set 4 reps / weight	Set 5 reps / weight
1. ☐	____X____	____X____	____X____	____X____	____X____
2. ☐	____X____	____X____	____X____	____X____	____X____
3. ☐	____X____	____X____	____X____	____X____	____X____
4. ☐	____X____	____X____	____X____	____X____	____X____
5. ☐	____X____	____X____	____X____	____X____	____X____
6. ☐	____X____	____X____	____X____	____X____	____X____
7. ☐	____X____	____X____	____X____	____X____	____X____
8. ☐	____X____	____X____	____X____	____X____	____X____
9. ☐	____X____	____X____	____X____	____X____	____X____
10. ☐	____X____	____X____	____X____	____X____	____X____
11. ☐	____X____	____X____	____X____	____X____	____X____
12.	____X____	____X____	____X____	____X____	____X____

Workout Comments:

Supplements:

Sleep (hrs): 1 2 3 4 5 6 7 8 9 10+   Workout Rating: 1 2 3 4 5 6 7 8 9 10

Date:_____   Partner/Trainer:_____

Time:_____   Injuries:_____
      start / finish

Location:_____   BP/RHR/WT:_____

☐ Warm-up ☐ Stretching ☐ Cool-down

Cardio / Class Phase

Focus:
☐ Fat Burn ☐ Random
☐ Interval ☐ Bootcamp
☐ Manual   ☐ Circuit

Type	Duration (min)	HR (min/max)	Dist / Floors	Intensity	Calories

Training Phase

Focus:
☐ Upper: _____
☐ Lower: _____
☐ Full/Combo: _____

Exercise	Set 1 (WU) reps / weight	Set 2 reps / weight	Set 3 reps / weight	Set 4 reps / weight	Set 5 reps / weight
1.	___X___	___X___	___X___	___X___	___X___
2.	___X___	___X___	___X___	___X___	___X___
3.	___X___	___X___	___X___	___X___	___X___
4.	___X___	___X___	___X___	___X___	___X___
5.	___X___	___X___	___X___	___X___	___X___
6.	___X___	___X___	___X___	___X___	___X___
7.	___X___	___X___	___X___	___X___	___X___
8.	___X___	___X___	___X___	___X___	___X___
9.	___X___	___X___	___X___	___X___	___X___
10.	___X___	___X___	___X___	___X___	___X___
11.	___X___	___X___	___X___	___X___	___X___
12.	___X___	___X___	___X___	___X___	___X___

Workout Comments:

Supplements:

Sleep (hrs): 1 2 3 4 5 6 7 8 9 10+   Workout Rating: 1 2 3 4 5 6 7 8 9 10

Partner/Trainer:_____

Injuries:_____

BP/RHR/WT:_____

Date:_____

Time:_____ start / finish

Location:_____

☐ Warm-up   ☐ Stretching   ☐ Cool-down

Cardio / Class Phase

Focus:
☐ Fat Burn   ☐ Random
☐ Interval   ☐ Bootcamp
☐ Manual   ☐ Circuit

Type	Duration (min)	HR (min/max)	Dist / Floors	Intensity	Calories

Training Phase

Focus:
☐ Upper: _____
☐ Lower: _____
☐ Full/Combo: _____

Exercise	Set 1 (WU) reps / weight	Set 2 reps / weight	Set 3 reps / weight	Set 4 reps / weight	Set 5 reps / weight
1.	____ x ____	____ x ____	____ x ____	____ x ____	____ x ____
2.	____ x ____	____ x ____	____ x ____	____ x ____	____ x ____
3.	____ x ____	____ x ____	____ x ____	____ x ____	____ x ____
4.	____ x ____	____ x ____	____ x ____	____ x ____	____ x ____
5.	____ x ____	____ x ____	____ x ____	____ x ____	____ x ____
6.	____ x ____	____ x ____	____ x ____	____ x ____	____ x ____
7.	____ x ____	____ x ____	____ x ____	____ x ____	____ x ____
8.	____ x ____	____ x ____	____ x ____	____ x ____	____ x ____
9.	____ x ____	____ x ____	____ x ____	____ x ____	____ x ____
10.	____ x ____	____ x ____	____ x ____	____ x ____	____ x ____
11.	____ x ____	____ x ____	____ x ____	____ x ____	____ x ____
12.	____ x ____	____ x ____	____ x ____	____ x ____	____ x ____

Workout Comments:

Supplements:

Sleep (hrs): 1 2 3 4 5 6 7 8 9 10+   Workout Rating: 1 2 3 4 5 6 7 8 9 10

Date:_____   Partner/Trainer:_____

Time:_____ start / finish   Injuries:_____

Location:_____   BP/RHR/WT:_____

☐ Warm-up   ☐ Stretching   ☐ Cool-down

Cardio / Class Phase   Focus:

☐ Fat Burn   ☐ Random
☐ Interval   ☐ Bootcamp
☐ Manual   ☐ Circuit

Type	Duration (min)	HR (min/max)	Dist / Floors	Intensity	Calories

Training Phase   Focus:

☐ Upper: _____
☐ Lower: _____
☐ Full/Combo: _____

Exercise	Set 1 (WU) reps / weight	Set 2 reps / weight	Set 3 reps / weight	Set 4 reps / weight	Set 5 reps / weight
1.	___X___	___X___	___X___	___X___	___X___
2.	___X___	___X___	___X___	___X___	___X___
3.	___X___	___X___	___X___	___X___	___X___
4.	___X___	___X___	___X___	___X___	___X___
5.	___X___	___X___	___X___	___X___	___X___
6.	___X___	___X___	___X___	___X___	___X___
7.	___X___	___X___	___X___	___X___	___X___
8.	___X___	___X___	___X___	___X___	___X___
9.	___X___	___X___	___X___	___X___	___X___
10.	___X___	___X___	___X___	___X___	___X___
11.	___X___	___X___	___X___	___X___	___X___
12.	___X___	___X___	___X___	___X___	___X___

Workout Comments:

Supplements:

Sleep (hrs): 1 2 3 4 5 6 7 8 9 10+   Workout Rating: 1 2 3 4 5 6 7 8 9 10

Partner/Trainer:_____

Injuries:_____

BP/RHR/WT:_____

Date:_____

Time:_____ start / finish

Location:_____

☐ Warm-up ☐ Stretching ☐ Cool-down

Cardio / Class Phase

Focus:

☐ Fat Burn ☐ Random
☐ Interval ☐ Bootcamp
☐ Manual ☐ Circuit

Type	Duration (min)	HR (min/max)	Dist / Floors	Intensity	Calories

Training Phase

Focus:

☐ Upper: _____
☐ Lower: _____
☐ Full/Combo: _____

Exercise	Set 1 (WU) reps / weight	Set 2 reps / weight	Set 3 reps / weight	Set 4 reps / weight	Set 5 reps / weight
1. ☐	___x___	___x___	___x___	___x___	___x___
2. ☐	___x___	___x___	___x___	___x___	___x___
3. ☐	___x___	___x___	___x___	___x___	___x___
4. ☐	___x___	___x___	___x___	___x___	___x___
5. ☐	___x___	___x___	___x___	___x___	___x___
6. ☐	___x___	___x___	___x___	___x___	___x___
7. ☐	___x___	___x___	___x___	___x___	___x___
8. ☐	___x___	___x___	___x___	___x___	___x___
9. ☐	___x___	___x___	___x___	___x___	___x___
10. ☐	___x___	___x___	___x___	___x___	___x___
11. ☐	___x___	___x___	___x___	___x___	___x___
12.	___x___	___x___	___x___	___x___	___x___

Workout Comments:

Supplements:

Sleep (hrs): 1 2 3 4 5 6 7 8 9 10+   Workout Rating: 1 2 3 4 5 6 7 8 9 10

Date:_____   Partner/Trainer:_____

Time:_____ start / finish   Injuries:_____

Location:_____   BP/RHR/WT:_____

☐ Warm-up   ☐ Stretching   ☐ Cool-down

Cardio / Class Phase

Focus:
☐ Fat Burn ☐ Random
☐ Interval ☐ Bootcamp
☐ Manual   ☐ Circuit

Type	Duration (min)	HR (min/max)	Dist / Floors	Intensity	Calories

Training Phase

Focus:
☐ Upper: _____
☐ Lower: _____
☐ Full/Combo: _____

Exercise	Set 1 (WU) reps / weight	Set 2 reps / weight	Set 3 reps / weight	Set 4 reps / weight	Set 5 reps / weight
1. ☐	___X___	___X___	___X___	___X___	___X___
2. ☐	___X___	___X___	___X___	___X___	___X___
3. ☐	___X___	___X___	___X___	___X___	___X___
4. ☐	___X___	___X___	___X___	___X___	___X___
5. ☐	___X___	___X___	___X___	___X___	___X___
6. ☐	___X___	___X___	___X___	___X___	___X___
7. ☐	___X___	___X___	___X___	___X___	___X___
8. ☐	___X___	___X___	___X___	___X___	___X___
9. ☐	___X___	___X___	___X___	___X___	___X___
10. ☐	___X___	___X___	___X___	___X___	___X___
11. ☐	___X___	___X___	___X___	___X___	___X___
12.	___X___	___X___	___X___	___X___	___X___

Workout Comments:

Supplements:

Sleep (hrs): 1 2 3 4 5 6 7 8 9 10+   **Workout Rating:** 1 2 3 4 5 6 7 8 9 10

Partner/Trainer:_____

Injuries:_____

BP/RHR/WT:_____

Date:_____

Time:_____ start / finish

Location:_____

☐ Warm-up   ☐ Stretching   ☐ Cool-down

Cardio / Class Phase   Focus:

☐ Fat Burn   ☐ Random
☐ Interval   ☐ Bootcamp
☐ Manual   ☐ Circuit

Type	Duration (min)	HR (min/max)	Dist / Floors	Intensity	Calories

Training Phase   Focus:

☐ Upper: _____
☐ Lower: _____
☐ Full/Combo: _____

Exercise	Set 1 (WU) reps / weight	Set 2 reps / weight	Set 3 reps / weight	Set 4 reps / weight	Set 5 reps / weight
1.	___X___	___X___	___X___	___X___	___X___
2.	___X___	___X___	___X___	___X___	___X___
3.	___X___	___X___	___X___	___X___	___X___
4.	___X___	___X___	___X___	___X___	___X___
5.	___X___	___X___	___X___	___X___	___X___
6.	___X___	___X___	___X___	___X___	___X___
7.	___X___	___X___	___X___	___X___	___X___
8.	___X___	___X___	___X___	___X___	___X___
9.	___X___	___X___	___X___	___X___	___X___
10.	___X___	___X___	___X___	___X___	___X___
11.	___X___	___X___	___X___	___X___	___X___
12.	___X___	___X___	___X___	___X___	___X___

Workout Comments:

Supplements:

Sleep (hrs): 1 2 3 4 5 6 7 8 9 10+   Workout Rating: 1 2 3 4 5 6 7 8 9 10

Date:_____ Partner/Trainer:_____

Time:_____ start / finish Injuries:_____

Location:_____ BP/RHR/WT:_____

☐ Warm-up ☐ Stretching ☐ Cool-down

Cardio / Class Phase

Focus:
☐ Fat Burn ☐ Random
☐ Interval ☐ Bootcamp
☐ Manual ☐ Circuit

Type	Duration (min)	HR (min/max)	Dist / Floors	Intensity	Calories

Training Phase

Focus:
☐ Upper: _____
☐ Lower: _____
☐ Full/Combo: _____

Exercise	Set 1 (WU) reps / weight	Set 2 reps / weight	Set 3 reps / weight	Set 4 reps / weight	Set 5 reps / weight
1.	___X___	___X___	___X___	___X___	___X___
2.	___X___	___X___	___X___	___X___	___X___
3.	___X___	___X___	___X___	___X___	___X___
4.	___X___	___X___	___X___	___X___	___X___
5.	___X___	___X___	___X___	___X___	___X___
6.	___X___	___X___	___X___	___X___	___X___
7.	___X___	___X___	___X___	___X___	___X___
8.	___X___	___X___	___X___	___X___	___X___
9.	___X___	___X___	___X___	___X___	___X___
10.	___X___	___X___	___X___	___X___	___X___
11.	___X___	___X___	___X___	___X___	___X___
12.	___X___	___X___	___X___	___X___	___X___

Workout Comments:

Supplements:

Sleep (hrs): 1 2 3 4 5 6 7 8 9 10+   Workout Rating: 1 2 3 4 5 6 7 8 9 10

Partner/Trainer:_____

Injuries:_____

BP/RHR/WT:_____

Date:_____

Time:_____ start / finish

Location:_____

☐ Warm-up   ☐ Stretching   ☐ Cool-down

Cardio / Class Phase

Focus:
☐ Fat Burn   ☐ Random
☐ Interval   ☐ Bootcamp
☐ Manual   ☐ Circuit

Type	Duration (min)	HR (min/max)	Dist / Floors	Intensity	Calories

Training Phase   **Focus:**
☐ Upper: _____
☐ Lower: _____
☐ Full/Combo: _____

Exercise	Set 1 (WU) reps / weight	Set 2 reps / weight	Set 3 reps / weight	Set 4 reps / weight	Set 5 reps / weight
1.	___X___	___X___	___X___	___X___	___X___
2.	___X___	___X___	___X___	___X___	___X___
3.	___X___	___X___	___X___	___X___	___X___
4.	___X___	___X___	___X___	___X___	___X___
5.	___X___	___X___	___X___	___X___	___X___
6.	___X___	___X___	___X___	___X___	___X___
7.	___X___	___X___	___X___	___X___	___X___
8.	___X___	___X___	___X___	___X___	___X___
9.	___X___	___X___	___X___	___X___	___X___
10.	___X___	___X___	___X___	___X___	___X___
11.	___X___	___X___	___X___	___X___	___X___
12.	___X___	___X___	___X___	___X___	___X___

Workout Comments:

Supplements:

Sleep (hrs): 1 2 3 4 5 6 7 8 9 10+   Workout Rating: 1 2 3 4 5 6 7 8 9 10

Date:_____   Partner/Trainer:_____

Time:_____ start / finish _____   Injuries:_____

Location:_____   BP/RHR/WT:_____

☐ Warm-up   ☐ Stretching   ☐ Cool-down

Cardio / Class Phase

Focus:
☐ Fat Burn   ☐ Random
☐ Interval   ☐ Bootcamp
☐ Manual   ☐ Circuit

Type	Duration (min)	HR (min/max)	Dist / Floors	Intensity	Calories

Training Phase

Focus:
☐ Upper: _____
☐ Lower: _____
☐ Full/Combo: _____

Exercise	Set 1 (WU) reps / weight	Set 2 reps / weight	Set 3 reps / weight	Set 4 reps / weight	Set 5 reps / weight
1. ☐	___X___	___X___	___X___	___X___	___X___
2. ☐	___X___	___X___	___X___	___X___	___X___
3. ☐	___X___	___X___	___X___	___X___	___X___
4. ☐	___X___	___X___	___X___	___X___	___X___
5. ☐	___X___	___X___	___X___	___X___	___X___
6. ☐	___X___	___X___	___X___	___X___	___X___
7. ☐	___X___	___X___	___X___	___X___	___X___
8. ☐	___X___	___X___	___X___	___X___	___X___
9. ☐	___X___	___X___	___X___	___X___	___X___
10. ☐	___X___	___X___	___X___	___X___	___X___
11. ☐	___X___	___X___	___X___	___X___	___X___
12.	___X___	___X___	___X___	___X___	___X___

Workout Comments:

Supplements:

Sleep (hrs): 1 2 3 4 5 6 7 8 9 10+   Workout Rating: 1 2 3 4 5 6 7 8 9 10

Partner/Trainer:_____

Injuries:_____

BP/RHR/WT:_____

Date:_____

Time:_____ start / finish

Location:_____

☐ Warm-up   ☐ Stretching   ☐ Cool-down

Cardio / Class Phase   Focus:

☐ Fat Burn   ☐ Random
☐ Interval   ☐ Bootcamp
☐ Manual   ☐ Circuit

Type	Duration (min)	HR (min/max)	Dist / Floors	Intensity	Calories

Training Phase   Focus:

☐ Upper: _____
☐ Lower: _____
☐ Full/Combo: _____

Exercise	Set 1 (WU) reps / weight	Set 2 reps / weight	Set 3 reps / weight	Set 4 reps / weight	Set 5 reps / weight
1.	___X___	___X___	___X___	___X___	___X___
2.	___X___	___X___	___X___	___X___	___X___
3.	___X___	___X___	___X___	___X___	___X___
4.	___X___	___X___	___X___	___X___	___X___
5.	___X___	___X___	___X___	___X___	___X___
6.	___X___	___X___	___X___	___X___	___X___
7.	___X___	___X___	___X___	___X___	___X___
8.	___X___	___X___	___X___	___X___	___X___
9.	___X___	___X___	___X___	___X___	___X___
10.	___X___	___X___	___X___	___X___	___X___
11.	___X___	___X___	___X___	___X___	___X___
12.	___X___	___X___	___X___	___X___	___X___

Workout Comments:

Supplements:

Sleep (hrs): 1 2 3 4 5 6 7 8 9 10+   Workout Rating: 1 2 3 4 5 6 7 8 9 10

Date:_____   Partner/Trainer:_____

Time:_____ start / finish _____   Injuries:_____

Location:_____   BP/RHR/WT:_____

☐ Warm-up   ☐ Stretching   ☐ Cool-down

Cardio / Class Phase   Focus:

☐ Fat Burn   ☐ Random
☐ Interval   ☐ Bootcamp
☐ Manual   ☐ Circuit

Type	Duration (min)	HR (min/max)	Dist / Floors	Intensity	Calories

Training Phase   Focus:

☐ Upper: _____
☐ Lower: _____
☐ Full/Combo: _____

Exercise	Set 1 (WU) reps / weight	Set 2 reps / weight	Set 3 reps / weight	Set 4 reps / weight	Set 5 reps / weight
1.	___ x ___	___ x ___	___ x ___	___ x ___	___ x ___
2.	___ x ___	___ x ___	___ x ___	___ x ___	___ x ___
3.	___ x ___	___ x ___	___ x ___	___ x ___	___ x ___
4.	___ x ___	___ x ___	___ x ___	___ x ___	___ x ___
5.	___ x ___	___ x ___	___ x ___	___ x ___	___ x ___
6.	___ x ___	___ x ___	___ x ___	___ x ___	___ x ___
7.	___ x ___	___ x ___	___ x ___	___ x ___	___ x ___
8.	___ x ___	___ x ___	___ x ___	___ x ___	___ x ___
9.	___ x ___	___ x ___	___ x ___	___ x ___	___ x ___
10.	___ x ___	___ x ___	___ x ___	___ x ___	___ x ___
11.	___ x ___	___ x ___	___ x ___	___ x ___	___ x ___
12.	___ x ___	___ x ___	___ x ___	___ x ___	___ x ___

Workout Comments:

Supplements:

Sleep (hrs): 1 2 3 4 5 6 7 8 9 10+   Workout Rating: 1 2 3 4 5 6 7 8 9 10

Partner/Trainer:_____

Injuries:_____

BP/RHR/WT:_____

Date:_____

Time:_____ start / finish

Location:_____

☐ Warm-up   ☐ Stretching   ☐ Cool-down

Cardio / Class Phase

Focus:
☐ Fat Burn   ☐ Random
☐ Interval   ☐ Bootcamp
☐ Manual   ☐ Circuit

Type	Duration (min)	HR (min/max)	Dist / Floors	Intensity	Calories

Training Phase

Focus:
☐ Upper: _____
☐ Lower: _____
☐ Full/Combo: _____

Exercise	Set 1 (WU) reps / weight	Set 2 reps / weight	Set 3 reps / weight	Set 4 reps / weight	Set 5 reps / weight
1.	___x___	___x___	___x___	___x___	___x___
2.	___x___	___x___	___x___	___x___	___x___
3.	___x___	___x___	___x___	___x___	___x___
4.	___x___	___x___	___x___	___x___	___x___
5.	___x___	___x___	___x___	___x___	___x___
6.	___x___	___x___	___x___	___x___	___x___
7.	___x___	___x___	___x___	___x___	___x___
8.	___x___	___x___	___x___	___x___	___x___
9.	___x___	___x___	___x___	___x___	___x___
10.	___x___	___x___	___x___	___x___	___x___
11.	___x___	___x___	___x___	___x___	___x___
12.	___x___	___x___	___x___	___x___	___x___

Workout Comments:

Supplements:

Sleep (hrs): 1 2 3 4 5 6 7 8 9 10+   Workout Rating: 1 2 3 4 5 6 7 8 9 10

Date:_____   Partner/Trainer:_____

Time:_____ start / finish _____   Injuries:_____

Location:_____   BP/RHR/WT:_____

☐ Warm-up ☐ Stretching ☐ Cool-down

Cardio / Class Phase

Focus:
☐ Fat Burn   ☐ Random
☐ Interval   ☐ Bootcamp
☐ Manual   ☐ Circuit

Type	Duration (min)	HR (min/max)	Dist / Floors	Intensity	Calories

Training Phase

Focus:
☐ Upper: _____
☐ Lower: _____
☐ Full/Combo: _____

Exercise	Set 1 (WU) reps / weight	Set 2 reps / weight	Set 3 reps / weight	Set 4 reps / weight	Set 5 reps / weight
1.	___X___	___X___	___X___	___X___	___X___
2.	___X___	___X___	___X___	___X___	___X___
3.	___X___	___X___	___X___	___X___	___X___
4.	___X___	___X___	___X___	___X___	___X___
5.	___X___	___X___	___X___	___X___	___X___
6.	___X___	___X___	___X___	___X___	___X___
7.	___X___	___X___	___X___	___X___	___X___
8.	___X___	___X___	___X___	___X___	___X___
9.	___X___	___X___	___X___	___X___	___X___
10.	___X___	___X___	___X___	___X___	___X___
11.	___X___	___X___	___X___	___X___	___X___
12.	___X___	___X___	___X___	___X___	___X___

Workout Comments:

Supplements:

Sleep (hrs): 1 2 3 4 5 6 7 8 9 10+   Workout Rating: 1 2 3 4 5 6 7 8 9 10

Partner/Trainer:_____

Injuries:_____

BP/RHR/WT:_____

Date:_____

Time:_____ start / finish

Location:_____

☐ Warm-up ☐ Stretching ☐ Cool-down

Cardio / Class Phase

Focus:
☐ Fat Burn ☐ Random
☐ Interval ☐ Bootcamp
☐ Manual ☐ Circuit

Type	Duration (min)	HR (min/max)	Dist / Floors	Intensity	Calories

Training Phase

Focus:
☐ Upper: _____
☐ Lower: _____
☐ Full/Combo: _____

Exercise	Set 1 (WU) reps / weight	Set 2 reps / weight	Set 3 reps / weight	Set 4 reps / weight	Set 5 reps / weight
1.	___x___	___x___	___x___	___x___	___x___
2.	___x___	___x___	___x___	___x___	___x___
3.	___x___	___x___	___x___	___x___	___x___
4.	___x___	___x___	___x___	___x___	___x___
5.	___x___	___x___	___x___	___x___	___x___
6.	___x___	___x___	___x___	___x___	___x___
7.	___x___	___x___	___x___	___x___	___x___
8.	___x___	___x___	___x___	___x___	___x___
9.	___x___	___x___	___x___	___x___	___x___
10.	___x___	___x___	___x___	___x___	___x___
11.	___x___	___x___	___x___	___x___	___x___
12.	___x___	___x___	___x___	___x___	___x___

Workout Comments:

Supplements:

Sleep (hrs): 1 2 3 4 5 6 7 8 9 10+   Workout Rating: 1 2 3 4 5 6 7 8 9 10

Date:_____   Partner/Trainer:_____

Time:_____   Injuries:_____
            start / finish
Location:_____   BP/RHR/WT:_____

☐ Warm-up   ☐ Stretching   ☐ Cool-down

Cardio / Class Phase   Focus:

☐ Fat Burn   ☐ Random
☐ Interval   ☐ Bootcamp
☐ Manual   ☐ Circuit

Type	Duration (min)	HR (min/max)	Dist / Floors	Intensity	Calories

Training Phase   Focus:

☐ Upper: _____
☐ Lower: _____
☐ Full/Combo: _____

Exercise	Set 1 (WU) reps / weight	Set 2 reps / weight	Set 3 reps / weight	Set 4 reps / weight	Set 5 reps / weight
1. ☐	___X___	___X___	___X___	___X___	___X___
2. ☐	___X___	___X___	___X___	___X___	___X___
3. ☐	___X___	___X___	___X___	___X___	___X___
4. ☐	___X___	___X___	___X___	___X___	___X___
5. ☐	___X___	___X___	___X___	___X___	___X___
6. ☐	___X___	___X___	___X___	___X___	___X___
7. ☐	___X___	___X___	___X___	___X___	___X___
8. ☐	___X___	___X___	___X___	___X___	___X___
9. ☐	___X___	___X___	___X___	___X___	___X___
10. ☐	___X___	___X___	___X___	___X___	___X___
11. ☐	___X___	___X___	___X___	___X___	___X___
12.	___X___	___X___	___X___	___X___	___X___

Workout Comments:

Supplements:

Sleep (hrs): 1 2 3 4 5 6 7 8 9 10+   Workout Rating: 1 2 3 4 5 6 7 8 9 10

Partner/Trainer:_____   Date:_____

Injuries:_____   Time:_____ start / finish _____

BP/RHR/WT:_____   Location:_____

☐ Warm-up   ☐ Stretching   ☐ Cool-down

Cardio / Class Phase   Focus:

☐ Fat Burn   ☐ Random
☐ Interval   ☐ Bootcamp
☐ Manual   ☐ Circuit

Type	Duration (min)	HR (min/max)	Dist / Floors	Intensity	Calories

Training Phase   Focus:

☐ Upper: _____
☐ Lower: _____
☐ Full/Combo: _____

Exercise	Set 1 (WU) reps / weight	Set 2 reps / weight	Set 3 reps / weight	Set 4 reps / weight	Set 5 reps / weight
1. ☐	___ X ___	___ X ___	___ X ___	___ X ___	___ X ___
2. ☐	___ X ___	___ X ___	___ X ___	___ X ___	___ X ___
3. ☐	___ X ___	___ X ___	___ X ___	___ X ___	___ X ___
4. ☐	___ X ___	___ X ___	___ X ___	___ X ___	___ X ___
5. ☐	___ X ___	___ X ___	___ X ___	___ X ___	___ X ___
6. ☐	___ X ___	___ X ___	___ X ___	___ X ___	___ X ___
7. ☐	___ X ___	___ X ___	___ X ___	___ X ___	___ X ___
8. ☐	___ X ___	___ X ___	___ X ___	___ X ___	___ X ___
9. ☐	___ X ___	___ X ___	___ X ___	___ X ___	___ X ___
10. ☐	___ X ___	___ X ___	___ X ___	___ X ___	___ X ___
11. ☐	___ X ___	___ X ___	___ X ___	___ X ___	___ X ___
12.	___ X ___	___ X ___	___ X ___	___ X ___	___ X ___

Workout Comments:

Supplements:

Sleep (hrs): 1 2 3 4 5 6 7 8 9 10+   Workout Rating: 1 2 3 4 5 6 7 8 9 10

Date:_____ Partner/Trainer:_____

Time:_____ Injuries:_____
          start / finish

Location:_____ BP/RHR/WT:_____

☐ Warm-up   ☐ Stretching   ☐ Cool-down

Cardio / Class Phase   Focus:
| | | | Focus | | |
☐ Fat Burn ☐ Random
☐ Interval ☐ Bootcamp
☐ Manual   ☐ Circuit

Type	Duration (min)	HR (min/max)	Dist / Floors	Intensity	Calories

Training Phase   Focus:
☐ Upper: _____
☐ Lower: _____
☐ Full/Combo: _____

Exercise	Set 1 (WU) reps / weight	Set 2 reps / weight	Set 3 reps / weight	Set 4 reps / weight	Set 5 reps / weight
1. ☐	___X___	___X___	___X___	___X___	___X___
2. ☐	___X___	___X___	___X___	___X___	___X___
3. ☐	___X___	___X___	___X___	___X___	___X___
4. ☐	___X___	___X___	___X___	___X___	___X___
5. ☐	___X___	___X___	___X___	___X___	___X___
6. ☐	___X___	___X___	___X___	___X___	___X___
7. ☐	___X___	___X___	___X___	___X___	___X___
8. ☐	___X___	___X___	___X___	___X___	___X___
9. ☐	___X___	___X___	___X___	___X___	___X___
10. ☐	___X___	___X___	___X___	___X___	___X___
11. ☐	___X___	___X___	___X___	___X___	___X___
12.	___X___	___X___	___X___	___X___	___X___

Workout Comments:

Supplements:

Sleep (hrs): 1 2 3 4 5 6 7 8 9 10+   Workout Rating: 1 2 3 4 5 6 7 8 9 10

Partner/Trainer:_____   Date:_____

Injuries:_____   Time:_____ start / finish _____

BP/RHR/WT:_____   Location:_____

☐ Warm-up   ☐ Stretching   ☐ Cool-down

Cardio / Class Phase   Focus:

☐ Fat Burn   ☐ Random
☐ Interval   ☐ Bootcamp
☐ Manual   ☐ Circuit

Type	Duration (min)	HR (min/max)	Dist / Floors	Intensity	Calories

Training Phase   Focus:

☐ Upper: _____
☐ Lower: _____
☐ Full/Combo: _____

Exercise	Set 1 (WU) reps / weight	Set 2 reps / weight	Set 3 reps / weight	Set 4 reps / weight	Set 5 reps / weight
1. ☐	___x___	___x___	___x___	___x___	___x___
2. ☐	___x___	___x___	___x___	___x___	___x___
3. ☐	___x___	___x___	___x___	___x___	___x___
4. ☐	___x___	___x___	___x___	___x___	___x___
5. ☐	___x___	___x___	___x___	___x___	___x___
6. ☐	___x___	___x___	___x___	___x___	___x___
7. ☐	___x___	___x___	___x___	___x___	___x___
8. ☐	___x___	___x___	___x___	___x___	___x___
9. ☐	___x___	___x___	___x___	___x___	___x___
10. ☐	___x___	___x___	___x___	___x___	___x___
11. ☐	___x___	___x___	___x___	___x___	___x___
12.	___x___	___x___	___x___	___x___	___x___

Workout Comments:

Supplements:

Sleep (hrs):   1   2   3   4   5   6   7   8   9   10+   Workout Rating: 1   2   3   4   5   6   7   8   9   10

Date:_____   Partner/Trainer:_____

Time:_____ start / finish   Injuries:_____

Location:_____   BP/RHR/WT:_____

☐ Warm-up ☐ Stretching ☐ Cool-down

Cardio / Class Phase

Focus:
☐ Fat Burn ☐ Random
☐ Interval ☐ Bootcamp
☐ Manual   ☐ Circuit

Type	Duration (min)	HR (min/max)	Dist / Floors	Intensity	Calories

Training Phase

Focus:
☐ Upper: _____
☐ Lower: _____
☐ Full/Combo: _____

Exercise	Set 1 (WU) reps / weight	Set 2 reps / weight	Set 3 reps / weight	Set 4 reps / weight	Set 5 reps / weight
1. ☐	___ X ___	___ X ___	___ X ___	___ X ___	___ X ___
2. ☐	___ X ___	___ X ___	___ X ___	___ X ___	___ X ___
3. ☐	___ X ___	___ X ___	___ X ___	___ X ___	___ X ___
4. ☐	___ X ___	___ X ___	___ X ___	___ X ___	___ X ___
5. ☐	___ X ___	___ X ___	___ X ___	___ X ___	___ X ___
6. ☐	___ X ___	___ X ___	___ X ___	___ X ___	___ X ___
7. ☐	___ X ___	___ X ___	___ X ___	___ X ___	___ X ___
8. ☐	___ X ___	___ X ___	___ X ___	___ X ___	___ X ___
9. ☐	___ X ___	___ X ___	___ X ___	___ X ___	___ X ___
10. ☐	___ X ___	___ X ___	___ X ___	___ X ___	___ X ___
11. ☐	___ X ___	___ X ___	___ X ___	___ X ___	___ X ___
12. ☐	___ X ___	___ X ___	___ X ___	___ X ___	___ X ___

Workout Comments:

Supplements:

Sleep (hrs): 1 2 3 4 5 6 7 8 9 10+   Workout Rating: 1 2 3 4 5 6 7 8 9 10

Partner/Trainer:_____ Date:_____

Injuries:_____ Time:_____ start / finish _____

BP/RHR/WT:_____ Location:_____

☐ Warm-up   ☐ Stretching   ☐ Cool-down

Cardio / Class Phase

Focus:
☐ Fat Burn   ☐ Random
☐ Interval   ☐ Bootcamp
☐ Manual   ☐ Circuit

Type	Duration (min)	HR (min/max)	Dist / Floors	Intensity	Calories

Training Phase

Focus:
☐ Upper: _____
☐ Lower: _____
☐ Full/Combo: _____

Exercise	Set 1 (WU) reps / weight	Set 2 reps / weight	Set 3 reps / weight	Set 4 reps / weight	Set 5 reps / weight
1. ☐	___ x ___	___ x ___	___ x ___	___ x ___	___ x ___
2. ☐	___ x ___	___ x ___	___ x ___	___ x ___	___ x ___
3. ☐	___ x ___	___ x ___	___ x ___	___ x ___	___ x ___
4. ☐	___ x ___	___ x ___	___ x ___	___ x ___	___ x ___
5. ☐	___ x ___	___ x ___	___ x ___	___ x ___	___ x ___
6. ☐	___ x ___	___ x ___	___ x ___	___ x ___	___ x ___
7. ☐	___ x ___	___ x ___	___ x ___	___ x ___	___ x ___
8. ☐	___ x ___	___ x ___	___ x ___	___ x ___	___ x ___
9. ☐	___ x ___	___ x ___	___ x ___	___ x ___	___ x ___
10. ☐	___ x ___	___ x ___	___ x ___	___ x ___	___ x ___
11. ☐	___ x ___	___ x ___	___ x ___	___ x ___	___ x ___
12.	___ x ___	___ x ___	___ x ___	___ x ___	___ x ___

Workout Comments:

Supplements:

Sleep (hrs): 1 2 3 4 5 6 7 8 9 10+   Workout Rating: 1 2 3 4 5 6 7 8 9 10

Date:_____   Partner/Trainer:_____

Time:_____ start / finish   Injuries:_____

Location:_____   BP/RHR/WT:_____

☐ Warm-up ☐ Stretching ☐ Cool-down

Cardio / Class Phase

Focus:
☐ Fat Burn ☐ Random
☐ Interval ☐ Bootcamp
☐ Manual ☐ Circuit

Type	Duration (min)	HR (min/max)	Dist / Floors	Intensity	Calories

Training Phase

Focus:
☐ Upper: _____
☐ Lower: _____
☐ Full/Combo: _____

Exercise	Set 1 (WU) reps / weight	Set 2 reps / weight	Set 3 reps / weight	Set 4 reps / weight	Set 5 reps / weight
1. ☐	___x___	___x___	___x___	___x___	___x___
2. ☐	___x___	___x___	___x___	___x___	___x___
3. ☐	___x___	___x___	___x___	___x___	___x___
4. ☐	___x___	___x___	___x___	___x___	___x___
5. ☐	___x___	___x___	___x___	___x___	___x___
6. ☐	___x___	___x___	___x___	___x___	___x___
7. ☐	___x___	___x___	___x___	___x___	___x___
8. ☐	___x___	___x___	___x___	___x___	___x___
9. ☐	___x___	___x___	___x___	___x___	___x___
10. ☐	___x___	___x___	___x___	___x___	___x___
11. ☐	___x___	___x___	___x___	___x___	___x___
12.	___x___	___x___	___x___	___x___	___x___

Workout Comments:

Supplements:

Sleep (hrs): 1 2 3 4 5 6 7 8 9 10+   Workout Rating: 1 2 3 4 5 6 7 8 9 10

Partner/Trainer:_____ Date:_____

Injuries:_____ Time:_____ start / finish _____

BP/RHR/WT:_____ Location:_____

☐ Warm-up   ☐ Stretching   ☐ Cool-down

Cardio / Class Phase   Focus:

☐ Fat Burn ☐ Random
☐ Interval ☐ Bootcamp
☐ Manual ☐ Circuit

Type	Duration (min)	HR (min/max)	Dist / Floors	Intensity	Calories

Training Phase   Focus:

☐ Upper: _____
☐ Lower: _____
☐ Full/Combo: _____

Exercise	Set 1 (WU) reps / weight	Set 2 reps / weight	Set 3 reps / weight	Set 4 reps / weight	Set 5 reps / weight
1.	____X____	____X____	____X____	____X____	____X____
2.	____X____	____X____	____X____	____X____	____X____
3.	____X____	____X____	____X____	____X____	____X____
4.	____X____	____X____	____X____	____X____	____X____
5.	____X____	____X____	____X____	____X____	____X____
6.	____X____	____X____	____X____	____X____	____X____
7.	____X____	____X____	____X____	____X____	____X____
8.	____X____	____X____	____X____	____X____	____X____
9.	____X____	____X____	____X____	____X____	____X____
10.	____X____	____X____	____X____	____X____	____X____
11.	____X____	____X____	____X____	____X____	____X____
12.	____X____	____X____	____X____	____X____	____X____

Workout Comments:

Supplements:

Sleep (hrs): 1 2 3 4 5 6 7 8 9 10+   Workout Rating: 1 2 3 4 5 6 7 8 9 10

Date:_____ Partner/Trainer:_____

Time:_____ Injuries:_____
     start / finish

Location:_____ BP/RHR/WT:_____

☐ Warm-up ☐ Stretching ☐ Cool-down

Cardio / Class Phase Focus:

☐ Fat Burn ☐ Random
☐ Interval ☐ Bootcamp
☐ Manual   ☐ Circuit

Type	Duration (min)	HR (min/max)	Dist / Floors	Intensity	Calories

Training Phase Focus:

☐ Upper: _____
☐ Lower: _____
☐ Full/Combo: _____

Exercise	Set 1 (WU) reps / weight	Set 2 reps / weight	Set 3 reps / weight	Set 4 reps / weight	Set 5 reps / weight
1. ☐	___X___	___X___	___X___	___X___	___X___
2. ☐	___X___	___X___	___X___	___X___	___X___
3. ☐	___X___	___X___	___X___	___X___	___X___
4. ☐	___X___	___X___	___X___	___X___	___X___
5. ☐	___X___	___X___	___X___	___X___	___X___
6. ☐	___X___	___X___	___X___	___X___	___X___
7. ☐	___X___	___X___	___X___	___X___	___X___
8. ☐	___X___	___X___	___X___	___X___	___X___
9. ☐	___X___	___X___	___X___	___X___	___X___
10. ☐	___X___	___X___	___X___	___X___	___X___
11. ☐	___X___	___X___	___X___	___X___	___X___
12.	___X___	___X___	___X___	___X___	___X___

Workout Comments:

Supplements:

Sleep (hrs): 1 2 3 4 5 6 7 8 9 10+   Workout Rating: 1 2 3 4 5 6 7 8 9 10

Partner/Trainer:_____ Date:_____

Injuries:_____ Time:_____ start / finish

BP/RHR/WT:_____ Location:_____

☐ Warm-up   ☐ Stretching   ☐ Cool-down

Cardio / Class Phase

Focus:
☐ Fat Burn   ☐ Random
☐ Interval   ☐ Bootcamp
☐ Manual   ☐ Circuit

Type	Duration (min)	HR (min/max)	Dist / Floors	Intensity	Calories

Training Phase

Focus:
☐ Upper: _____
☐ Lower: _____
☐ Full/Combo: _____

Exercise	Set 1 (WU) reps / weight	Set 2 reps / weight	Set 3 reps / weight	Set 4 reps / weight	Set 5 reps / weight
1.	___X___	___X___	___X___	___X___	___X___
2.	___X___	___X___	___X___	___X___	___X___
3.	___X___	___X___	___X___	___X___	___X___
4.	___X___	___X___	___X___	___X___	___X___
5.	___X___	___X___	___X___	___X___	___X___
6.	___X___	___X___	___X___	___X___	___X___
7.	___X___	___X___	___X___	___X___	___X___
8.	___X___	___X___	___X___	___X___	___X___
9.	___X___	___X___	___X___	___X___	___X___
10.	___X___	___X___	___X___	___X___	___X___
11.	___X___	___X___	___X___	___X___	___X___
12.	___X___	___X___	___X___	___X___	___X___

Workout Comments:

Supplements:

Sleep (hrs): 1 2 3 4 5 6 7 8 9 10+   Workout Rating: 1 2 3 4 5 6 7 8 9 10

Date:_____ Partner/Trainer:_____

Time:_____ Injuries:_____
       start / finish

Location:_____ BP/RHR/WT:_____

☐ Warm-up ☐ Stretching ☐ Cool-down

Cardio / Class Phase

Focus:
☐ Fat Burn ☐ Random
☐ Interval ☐ Bootcamp
☐ Manual   ☐ Circuit

Type	Duration (min)	HR (min/max)	Dist / Floors	Intensity	Calories

Training Phase

Focus:
☐ Upper: _____
☐ Lower: _____
☐ Full/Combo: _____

Exercise	Set 1 (WU) reps / weight	Set 2 reps / weight	Set 3 reps / weight	Set 4 reps / weight	Set 5 reps / weight
1.	___X___	___X___	___X___	___X___	___X___
2.	___X___	___X___	___X___	___X___	___X___
3.	___X___	___X___	___X___	___X___	___X___
4.	___X___	___X___	___X___	___X___	___X___
5.	___X___	___X___	___X___	___X___	___X___
6.	___X___	___X___	___X___	___X___	___X___
7.	___X___	___X___	___X___	___X___	___X___
8.	___X___	___X___	___X___	___X___	___X___
9.	___X___	___X___	___X___	___X___	___X___
10.	___X___	___X___	___X___	___X___	___X___
11.	___X___	___X___	___X___	___X___	___X___
12.	___X___	___X___	___X___	___X___	___X___

Workout Comments:

Supplements:

Sleep (hrs): 1 2 3 4 5 6 7 8 9 10+   Workout Rating: 1 2 3 4 5 6 7 8 9 10

Partner/Trainer:_____ Date:_____

Injuries:_____ Time:_____ start / finish _____

BP/RHR/WT:_____ Location:_____

☐ Warm-up ☐ Stretching ☐ Cool-down

Cardio / Class Phase

Focus:
☐ Fat Burn ☐ Random
☐ Interval ☐ Bootcamp
☐ Manual ☐ Circuit

Type	Duration (min)	HR (min/max)	Dist / Floors	Intensity	Calories

Training Phase

Focus:
☐ Upper: _____
☐ Lower: _____
☐ Full/Combo: _____

Exercise	Set 1 (WU) reps / weight	Set 2 reps / weight	Set 3 reps / weight	Set 4 reps / weight	Set 5 reps / weight
1. ☐	___ X ___	___ X ___	___ X ___	___ X ___	___ X ___
2. ☐	___ X ___	___ X ___	___ X ___	___ X ___	___ X ___
3. ☐	___ X ___	___ X ___	___ X ___	___ X ___	___ X ___
4. ☐	___ X ___	___ X ___	___ X ___	___ X ___	___ X ___
5. ☐	___ X ___	___ X ___	___ X ___	___ X ___	___ X ___
6. ☐	___ X ___	___ X ___	___ X ___	___ X ___	___ X ___
7. ☐	___ X ___	___ X ___	___ X ___	___ X ___	___ X ___
8. ☐	___ X ___	___ X ___	___ X ___	___ X ___	___ X ___
9. ☐	___ X ___	___ X ___	___ X ___	___ X ___	___ X ___
10. ☐	___ X ___	___ X ___	___ X ___	___ X ___	___ X ___
11. ☐	___ X ___	___ X ___	___ X ___	___ X ___	___ X ___
12. ☐	___ X ___	___ X ___	___ X ___	___ X ___	___ X ___

Workout Comments:

Supplements:

Sleep (hrs): 1 2 3 4 5 6 7 8 9 10+   Workout Rating: 1 2 3 4 5 6 7 8 9 10

Date:_____ Partner/Trainer:_____

Time:_____ start / finish _____ Injuries:_____

Location:_____ BP/RHR/WT:_____

□ Warm-up □ Stretching □ Cool-down

Cardio / Class Phase Focus:

□ Fat Burn □ Random
□ Interval □ Bootcamp
□ Manual □ Circuit

Type	Duration (min)	HR (min/max)	Dist / Floors	Intensity	Calories

Training Phase Focus:

□ Upper: _____
□ Lower: _____
□ Full/Combo: _____

Exercise	Set 1 (WU) reps / weight	Set 2 reps / weight	Set 3 reps / weight	Set 4 reps / weight	Set 5 reps / weight
1.	___X___	___X___	___X___	___X___	___X___
2.	___X___	___X___	___X___	___X___	___X___
3.	___X___	___X___	___X___	___X___	___X___
4.	___X___	___X___	___X___	___X___	___X___
5.	___X___	___X___	___X___	___X___	___X___
6.	___X___	___X___	___X___	___X___	___X___
7.	___X___	___X___	___X___	___X___	___X___
8.	___X___	___X___	___X___	___X___	___X___
9.	___X___	___X___	___X___	___X___	___X___
10.	___X___	___X___	___X___	___X___	___X___
11.	___X___	___X___	___X___	___X___	___X___
12.	___X___	___X___	___X___	___X___	___X___

Workout Comments:

Supplements:

Sleep (hrs): 1 2 3 4 5 6 7 8 9 10+   Workout Rating: 1 2 3 4 5 6 7 8 9 10

Partner/Trainer:_____

Injuries:_____

BP/RHR/WT:_____

Date:_____

Time:_____ start / finish _____

Location:_____

☐ Warm-up ☐ Stretching ☐ Cool-down

Cardio / Class Phase

Focus:
☐ Fat Burn ☐ Random
☐ Interval ☐ Bootcamp
☐ Manual ☐ Circuit

Type	Duration (min)	HR (min/max)	Dist / Floors	Intensity	Calories

Training Phase

Focus:
☐ Upper: _____
☐ Lower: _____
☐ Full/Combo: _____

Exercise	Set 1 (WU) reps / weight	Set 2 reps / weight	Set 3 reps / weight	Set 4 reps / weight	Set 5 reps / weight
1. ☐	___X___	___X___	___X___	___X___	___X___
2. ☐	___X___	___X___	___X___	___X___	___X___
3. ☐	___X___	___X___	___X___	___X___	___X___
4. ☐	___X___	___X___	___X___	___X___	___X___
5. ☐	___X___	___X___	___X___	___X___	___X___
6. ☐	___X___	___X___	___X___	___X___	___X___
7. ☐	___X___	___X___	___X___	___X___	___X___
8. ☐	___X___	___X___	___X___	___X___	___X___
9. ☐	___X___	___X___	___X___	___X___	___X___
10. ☐	___X___	___X___	___X___	___X___	___X___
11. ☐	___X___	___X___	___X___	___X___	___X___
12.	___X___	___X___	___X___	___X___	___X___

Workout Comments:

Supplements:

Sleep (hrs): 1 2 3 4 5 6 7 8 9 10+   Workout Rating: 1 2 3 4 5 6 7 8 9 10

Date:_____ Partner/Trainer:_____

Time:_____ start / finish Injuries:_____

Location:_____ BP/RHR/WT:_____

☐ Warm-up ☐ Stretching ☐ Cool-down

Cardio / Class Phase

Focus:
☐ Fat Burn ☐ Random
☐ Interval ☐ Bootcamp
☐ Manual ☐ Circuit

Type	Duration (min)	HR (min/max)	Dist / Floors	Intensity	Calories

Training Phase

Focus:
☐ Upper: _____
☐ Lower: _____
☐ Full/Combo: _____

Exercise	Set 1 (WU) reps / weight	Set 2 reps / weight	Set 3 reps / weight	Set 4 reps / weight	Set 5 reps / weight
1. ☐	___x___	___x___	___x___	___x___	___x___
2. ☐	___x___	___x___	___x___	___x___	___x___
3. ☐	___x___	___x___	___x___	___x___	___x___
4. ☐	___x___	___x___	___x___	___x___	___x___
5. ☐	___x___	___x___	___x___	___x___	___x___
6. ☐	___x___	___x___	___x___	___x___	___x___
7. ☐	___x___	___x___	___x___	___x___	___x___
8. ☐	___x___	___x___	___x___	___x___	___x___
9. ☐	___x___	___x___	___x___	___x___	___x___
10. ☐	___x___	___x___	___x___	___x___	___x___
11. ☐	___x___	___x___	___x___	___x___	___x___
12.	___x___	___x___	___x___	___x___	___x___

Workout Comments:

Supplements:

Sleep (hrs): 1 2 3 4 5 6 7 8 9 10+   Workout Rating: 1 2 3 4 5 6 7 8 9 10

Partner/Trainer:_____ Date:_____

Injuries:_____ Time:_____ start / finish _____

BP/RHR/WT:_____ Location:_____

☐ Warm-up ☐ Stretching ☐ Cool-down

Cardio / Class Phase   Focus:

☐ Fat Burn ☐ Random
☐ Interval ☐ Bootcamp
☐ Manual ☐ Circuit

Type	Duration (min)	HR (min/max)	Dist / Floors	Intensity	Calories

Training Phase   Focus:

☐ Upper: _____
☐ Lower: _____
☐ Full/Combo: _____

Exercise	Set 1 (WU) reps / weight	Set 2 reps / weight	Set 3 reps / weight	Set 4 reps / weight	Set 5 reps / weight
1.	___X___	___X___	___X___	___X___	___X___
2.	___X___	___X___	___X___	___X___	___X___
3.	___X___	___X___	___X___	___X___	___X___
4.	___X___	___X___	___X___	___X___	___X___
5.	___X___	___X___	___X___	___X___	___X___
6.	___X___	___X___	___X___	___X___	___X___
7.	___X___	___X___	___X___	___X___	___X___
8.	___X___	___X___	___X___	___X___	___X___
9.	___X___	___X___	___X___	___X___	___X___
10.	___X___	___X___	___X___	___X___	___X___
11.	___X___	___X___	___X___	___X___	___X___
12.	___X___	___X___	___X___	___X___	___X___

Workout Comments:

Supplements:

Sleep (hrs): 1 2 3 4 5 6 7 8 9 10+   Workout Rating: 1 2 3 4 5 6 7 8 9 10

Date:_____   Partner/Trainer:_____

Time:_____ start / finish _____   Injuries:_____

Location:_____   BP/RHR/WT:_____

☐ Warm-up ☐ Stretching ☐ Cool-down

Cardio / Class Phase   **Focus**:

☐ Fat Burn ☐ Random
☐ Interval ☐ Bootcamp
☐ Manual   ☐ Circuit

Type	Duration (min)	HR (min/max)	Dist / Floors	Intensity	Calories

Training Phase   **Focus**:

☐ Upper: _____
☐ Lower: _____
☐ Full/Combo: _____

Exercise	Set 1 (WU) reps / weight	Set 2 reps / weight	Set 3 reps / weight	Set 4 reps / weight	Set 5 reps / weight
1. ☐	____ x ____	____ x ____	____ x ____	____ x ____	____ x ____
2. ☐	____ x ____	____ x ____	____ x ____	____ x ____	____ x ____
3. ☐	____ x ____	____ x ____	____ x ____	____ x ____	____ x ____
4. ☐	____ x ____	____ x ____	____ x ____	____ x ____	____ x ____
5. ☐	____ x ____	____ x ____	____ x ____	____ x ____	____ x ____
6. ☐	____ x ____	____ x ____	____ x ____	____ x ____	____ x ____
7. ☐	____ x ____	____ x ____	____ x ____	____ x ____	____ x ____
8. ☐	____ x ____	____ x ____	____ x ____	____ x ____	____ x ____
9. ☐	____ x ____	____ x ____	____ x ____	____ x ____	____ x ____
10. ☐	____ x ____	____ x ____	____ x ____	____ x ____	____ x ____
11. ☐	____ x ____	____ x ____	____ x ____	____ x ____	____ x ____
12.	____ x ____	____ x ____	____ x ____	____ x ____	____ x ____

Workout Comments:

Supplements:

Sleep (hrs): 1 2 3 4 5 6 7 8 9 10+   Workout Rating: 1 2 3 4 5 6 7 8 9 10

Partner/Trainer:_____

Injuries:_____

BP/RHR/WT:_____

Date:_____

Time:_____ start / finish

Location:_____

☐ Warm-up   ☐ Stretching   ☐ Cool-down

Cardio / Class Phase

Focus:
☐ Fat Burn   ☐ Random
☐ Interval   ☐ Bootcamp
☐ Manual   ☐ Circuit

Type	Duration (min)	HR (min/max)	Dist / Floors	Intensity	Calories

Training Phase

Focus:
☐ Upper: _____
☐ Lower: _____
☐ Full/Combo: _____

Exercise	Set 1 (WU) reps / weight	Set 2 reps / weight	Set 3 reps / weight	Set 4 reps / weight	Set 5 reps / weight
1. ☐	__x__	__x__	__x__	__x__	__x__
2. ☐	__x__	__x__	__x__	__x__	__x__
3. ☐	__x__	__x__	__x__	__x__	__x__
4. ☐	__x__	__x__	__x__	__x__	__x__
5. ☐	__x__	__x__	__x__	__x__	__x__
6. ☐	__x__	__x__	__x__	__x__	__x__
7. ☐	__x__	__x__	__x__	__x__	__x__
8. ☐	__x__	__x__	__x__	__x__	__x__
9. ☐	__x__	__x__	__x__	__x__	__x__
10. ☐	__x__	__x__	__x__	__x__	__x__
11. ☐	__x__	__x__	__x__	__x__	__x__
12.	__x__	__x__	__x__	__x__	__x__

Workout Comments:

Supplements:

Sleep (hrs): 1 2 3 4 5 6 7 8 9 10+   Workout Rating: 1 2 3 4 5 6 7 8 9 10

Date:_____   Partner/Trainer:_____

Time:_____ start / finish   Injuries:_____

Location:_____   BP/RHR/WT:_____

☐ Warm-up ☐ Stretching ☐ Cool-down

Cardio / Class Phase   Focus:

☐ Fat Burn ☐ Random
☐ Interval ☐ Bootcamp
☐ Manual   ☐ Circuit

Type	Duration (min)	HR (min/max)	Dist / Floors	Intensity	Calories

Training Phase   Focus:

☐ Upper: _____
☐ Lower: _____
☐ Full/Combo: _____

Exercise	Set 1 (WU) reps / weight	Set 2 reps / weight	Set 3 reps / weight	Set 4 reps / weight	Set 5 reps / weight
1. ☐	__X__	__X__	__X__	__X__	__X__
2. ☐	__X__	__X__	__X__	__X__	__X__
3. ☐	__X__	__X__	__X__	__X__	__X__
4. ☐	__X__	__X__	__X__	__X__	__X__
5. ☐	__X__	__X__	__X__	__X__	__X__
6. ☐	__X__	__X__	__X__	__X__	__X__
7. ☐	__X__	__X__	__X__	__X__	__X__
8. ☐	__X__	__X__	__X__	__X__	__X__
9. ☐	__X__	__X__	__X__	__X__	__X__
10. ☐	__X__	__X__	__X__	__X__	__X__
11. ☐	__X__	__X__	__X__	__X__	__X__
12.	__X__	__X__	__X__	__X__	__X__

Workout Comments:

Supplements:

Sleep (hrs): 1 2 3 4 5 6 7 8 9 10+   Workout Rating: 1 2 3 4 5 6 7 8 9 10

Partner/Trainer:_____

Injuries:_____

BP/RHR/WT:_____

Date:_____

Time:_____ start / finish

Location:_____

☐ Warm-up   ☐ Stretching   ☐ Cool-down

Cardio / Class Phase

Focus:
☐ Fat Burn ☐ Random
☐ Interval ☐ Bootcamp
☐ Manual ☐ Circuit

Type	Duration (min)	HR (min/max)	Dist / Floors	Intensity	Calories

Training Phase

Focus:
☐ Upper: _____
☐ Lower: _____
☐ Full/Combo: _____

Exercise	Set 1 (WU) reps / weight	Set 2 reps / weight	Set 3 reps / weight	Set 4 reps / weight	Set 5 reps / weight
1.	___X___	___X___	___X___	___X___	___X___
2.	___X___	___X___	___X___	___X___	___X___
3.	___X___	___X___	___X___	___X___	___X___
4.	___X___	___X___	___X___	___X___	___X___
5.	___X___	___X___	___X___	___X___	___X___
6.	___X___	___X___	___X___	___X___	___X___
7.	___X___	___X___	___X___	___X___	___X___
8.	___X___	___X___	___X___	___X___	___X___
9.	___X___	___X___	___X___	___X___	___X___
10.	___X___	___X___	___X___	___X___	___X___
11.	___X___	___X___	___X___	___X___	___X___
12.	___X___	___X___	___X___	___X___	___X___

Workout Comments:

Supplements:

Sleep (hrs): 1 2 3 4 5 6 7 8 9 10+   Workout Rating: 1 2 3 4 5 6 7 8 9 10

Date:_____   Partner/Trainer:_____

Time:_____   Injuries:_____

      start / finish

Location:_____   BP/RHR/WT:_____

□ Warm-up   □ Stretching   □ Cool-down

Cardio / Class Phase   Focus:

□ Fat Burn   □ Random
□ Interval   □ Bootcamp
□ Manual   □ Circuit

Type	Duration (min)	HR (min/max)	Dist / Floors	Intensity	Calories

Training Phase   Focus:

□ Upper: _____
□ Lower: _____
□ Full/Combo: _____

Exercise	Set 1 (WU) reps / weight	Set 2 reps / weight	Set 3 reps / weight	Set 4 reps / weight	Set 5 reps / weight
1.	___x___	___x___	___x___	___x___	___x___
2.	___x___	___x___	___x___	___x___	___x___
3.	___x___	___x___	___x___	___x___	___x___
4.	___x___	___x___	___x___	___x___	___x___
5.	___x___	___x___	___x___	___x___	___x___
6.	___x___	___x___	___x___	___x___	___x___
7.	___x___	___x___	___x___	___x___	___x___
8.	___x___	___x___	___x___	___x___	___x___
9.	___x___	___x___	___x___	___x___	___x___
10.	___x___	___x___	___x___	___x___	___x___
11.	___x___	___x___	___x___	___x___	___x___
12.	___x___	___x___	___x___	___x___	___x___

Workout Comments:

Supplements:

Sleep (hrs):   1   2   3   4   5   6   7   8   9   10+   Workout Rating: 1   2   3   4   5   6   7   8   9   10

Partner/Trainer:_____
Injuries:_____
BP/RHR/WT:_____

Date:_____
Time:_____ start / finish
Location:_____

☐ Warm-up ☐ Stretching ☐ Cool-down

Cardio / Class Phase   Focus:

☐ Fat Burn   ☐ Random
☐ Interval   ☐ Bootcamp
☐ Manual   ☐ Circuit

Type	Duration (min)	HR (min/max)	Dist / Floors	Intensity	Calories

Training Phase   Focus:

☐ Upper: _____
☐ Lower: _____
☐ Full/Combo: _____

Exercise	Set 1 (WU) reps / weight	Set 2 reps / weight	Set 3 reps / weight	Set 4 reps / weight	Set 5 reps / weight
1. ☐	___X___	___X___	___X___	___X___	___X___
2. ☐	___X___	___X___	___X___	___X___	___X___
3. ☐	___X___	___X___	___X___	___X___	___X___
4. ☐	___X___	___X___	___X___	___X___	___X___
5. ☐	___X___	___X___	___X___	___X___	___X___
6. ☐	___X___	___X___	___X___	___X___	___X___
7. ☐	___X___	___X___	___X___	___X___	___X___
8. ☐	___X___	___X___	___X___	___X___	___X___
9. ☐	___X___	___X___	___X___	___X___	___X___
10. ☐	___X___	___X___	___X___	___X___	___X___
11. ☐	___X___	___X___	___X___	___X___	___X___
12.	___X___	___X___	___X___	___X___	___X___

Workout Comments:

Supplements:

Sleep (hrs): 1 2 3 4 5 6 7 8 9 10+   Workout Rating: 1 2 3 4 5 6 7 8 9 10

Date:_____ Partner/Trainer:_____
Time:___ start / finish ___ Injuries:_____
Location:_____ BP/RHR/WT:_____

☐ Warm-up ☐ Stretching ☐ Cool-down

Cardio / Class Phase Focus:
☐ Fat Burn ☐ Random
☐ Interval ☐ Bootcamp
☐ Manual ☐ Circuit

Type	Duration (min)	HR (min/max)	Dist / Floors	Intensity	Calories

Training Phase Focus:
☐ Upper: _____
☐ Lower: _____
☐ Full/Combo: _____

Exercise	Set 1 (WU) reps / weight	Set 2 reps / weight	Set 3 reps / weight	Set 4 reps / weight	Set 5 reps / weight
1.	___x___	___x___	___x___	___x___	___x___
2.	___x___	___x___	___x___	___x___	___x___
3.	___x___	___x___	___x___	___x___	___x___
4.	___x___	___x___	___x___	___x___	___x___
5.	___x___	___x___	___x___	___x___	___x___
6.	___x___	___x___	___x___	___x___	___x___
7.	___x___	___x___	___x___	___x___	___x___
8.	___x___	___x___	___x___	___x___	___x___
9.	___x___	___x___	___x___	___x___	___x___
10.	___x___	___x___	___x___	___x___	___x___
11.	___x___	___x___	___x___	___x___	___x___
12.	___x___	___x___	___x___	___x___	___x___

Workout Comments:

Supplements:

Sleep (hrs): 1 2 3 4 5 6 7 8 9 10+   Workout Rating: 1 2 3 4 5 6 7 8 9 10

Partner/Trainer:_____   Date:_____

Injuries:_____   Time:_____ start / finish

BP/RHR/WT:_____   Location:_____

☐ Warm-up   ☐ Stretching   ☐ Cool-down

Cardio / Class Phase

Focus:
☐ Fat Burn   ☐ Random
☐ Interval   ☐ Bootcamp
☐ Manual   ☐ Circuit

Type	Duration (min)	HR (min/max)	Dist / Floors	Intensity	Calories

Training Phase

Focus:
☐ Upper: _____
☐ Lower: _____
☐ Full/Combo: _____

Exercise	Set 1 (WU) reps / weight	Set 2 reps / weight	Set 3 reps / weight	Set 4 reps / weight	Set 5 reps / weight
1. ☐	___X___	___X___	___X___	___X___	___X___
2. ☐	___X___	___X___	___X___	___X___	___X___
3. ☐	___X___	___X___	___X___	___X___	___X___
4. ☐	___X___	___X___	___X___	___X___	___X___
5. ☐	___X___	___X___	___X___	___X___	___X___
6. ☐	___X___	___X___	___X___	___X___	___X___
7. ☐	___X___	___X___	___X___	___X___	___X___
8. ☐	___X___	___X___	___X___	___X___	___X___
9. ☐	___X___	___X___	___X___	___X___	___X___
10. ☐	___X___	___X___	___X___	___X___	___X___
11. ☐	___X___	___X___	___X___	___X___	___X___
12.	___X___	___X___	___X___	___X___	___X___

Workout Comments:

Supplements:

Sleep (hrs): 1 2 3 4 5 6 7 8 9 10+   Workout Rating: 1 2 3 4 5 6 7 8 9 10

Date:_____ Partner/Trainer:_____

Time:_____ start / finish Injuries:_____

Location:_____ BP/RHR/WT:_____

☐ Warm-up ☐ Stretching ☐ Cool-down

Cardio / Class Phase Focus:

☐ Fat Burn ☐ Random
☐ Interval ☐ Bootcamp
☐ Manual ☐ Circuit

Type	Duration (min)	HR (min/max)	Dist / Floors	Intensity	Calories

Training Phase Focus:

☐ Upper: _____
☐ Lower: _____
☐ Full/Combo: _____

Exercise	Set 1 (WU) reps / weight	Set 2 reps / weight	Set 3 reps / weight	Set 4 reps / weight	Set 5 reps / weight
1. ☐	___X___	___X___	___X___	___X___	___X___
2. ☐	___X___	___X___	___X___	___X___	___X___
3. ☐	___X___	___X___	___X___	___X___	___X___
4. ☐	___X___	___X___	___X___	___X___	___X___
5. ☐	___X___	___X___	___X___	___X___	___X___
6. ☐	___X___	___X___	___X___	___X___	___X___
7. ☐	___X___	___X___	___X___	___X___	___X___
8. ☐	___X___	___X___	___X___	___X___	___X___
9. ☐	___X___	___X___	___X___	___X___	___X___
10. ☐	___X___	___X___	___X___	___X___	___X___
11. ☐	___X___	___X___	___X___	___X___	___X___
12.	___X___	___X___	___X___	___X___	___X___

Workout Comments:

Supplements:

Sleep (hrs): 1 2 3 4 5 6 7 8 9 10+   Workout Rating: 1 2 3 4 5 6 7 8 9 10

Partner/Trainer:_____ Date:_____

Injuries:_____ Time:_____ start / finish

BP/RHR/WT:_____ Location:_____

☐ Warm-up   ☐ Stretching   ☐ Cool-down

Cardio / Class Phase

Focus:
☐ Fat Burn ☐ Random
☐ Interval ☐ Bootcamp
☐ Manual   ☐ Circuit

Type	Duration (min)	HR (min/max)	Dist / Floors	Intensity	Calories

Training Phase

Focus:
☐ Upper: _____
☐ Lower: _____
☐ Full/Combo: _____

Exercise	Set 1 (WU) reps / weight	Set 2 reps / weight	Set 3 reps / weight	Set 4 reps / weight	Set 5 reps / weight
1.	___x___	___x___	___x___	___x___	___x___
2.	___x___	___x___	___x___	___x___	___x___
3.	___x___	___x___	___x___	___x___	___x___
4.	___x___	___x___	___x___	___x___	___x___
5.	___x___	___x___	___x___	___x___	___x___
6.	___x___	___x___	___x___	___x___	___x___
7.	___x___	___x___	___x___	___x___	___x___
8.	___x___	___x___	___x___	___x___	___x___
9.	___x___	___x___	___x___	___x___	___x___
10.	___x___	___x___	___x___	___x___	___x___
11.	___x___	___x___	___x___	___x___	___x___
12.	___x___	___x___	___x___	___x___	___x___

Workout Comments:

Supplements:

Sleep (hrs): 1 2 3 4 5 6 7 8 9 10+   Workout Rating: 1 2 3 4 5 6 7 8 9 10

Date:_____   Partner/Trainer:_____

Time:_____ start / finish _____   Injuries:_____

Location:_____   BP/RHR/WT:_____

☐ Warm-up   ☐ Stretching   ☐ Cool-down

Cardio / Class Phase

Focus:
☐ Fat Burn   ☐ Random
☐ Interval   ☐ Bootcamp
☐ Manual   ☐ Circuit

Type	Duration (min)	HR (min/max)	Dist / Floors	Intensity	Calories

Training Phase

Focus:
☐ Upper:_____
☐ Lower:_____
☐ Full/Combo:_____

Exercise	Set 1 (WU) reps / weight	Set 2 reps / weight	Set 3 reps / weight	Set 4 reps / weight	Set 5 reps / weight
1.	__X__	__X__	__X__	__X__	__X__
2.	__X__	__X__	__X__	__X__	__X__
3.	__X__	__X__	__X__	__X__	__X__
4.	__X__	__X__	__X__	__X__	__X__
5.	__X__	__X__	__X__	__X__	__X__
6.	__X__	__X__	__X__	__X__	__X__
7.	__X__	__X__	__X__	__X__	__X__
8.	__X__	__X__	__X__	__X__	__X__
9.	__X__	__X__	__X__	__X__	__X__
10.	__X__	__X__	__X__	__X__	__X__
11.	__X__	__X__	__X__	__X__	__X__
12.	__X__	__X__	__X__	__X__	__X__

Workout Comments:

Supplements:

Sleep (hrs): 1 2 3 4 5 6 7 8 9 10+   Workout Rating: 1 2 3 4 5 6 7 8 9 10

Partner/Trainer:_____   Date:_____

Injuries:_____   Time:_____ start / finish

BP/RHR/WT:_____   Location:_____

☐ Warm-up   ☐ Stretching   ☐ Cool-down

Cardio / Class Phase

Focus: ☐ Fat Burn ☐ Random
☐ Interval ☐ Bootcamp
☐ Manual ☐ Circuit

Type	Duration (min)	HR (min/max)	Dist / Floors	Intensity	Calories

Training Phase

Focus: ☐ Upper: _____
☐ Lower: _____
☐ Full/Combo: _____

Exercise	Set 1 (WU) reps / weight	Set 2 reps / weight	Set 3 reps / weight	Set 4 reps / weight	Set 5 reps / weight
1. ☐	___x___	___x___	___x___	___x___	___x___
2. ☐	___x___	___x___	___x___	___x___	___x___
3. ☐	___x___	___x___	___x___	___x___	___x___
4. ☐	___x___	___x___	___x___	___x___	___x___
5. ☐	___x___	___x___	___x___	___x___	___x___
6. ☐	___x___	___x___	___x___	___x___	___x___
7. ☐	___x___	___x___	___x___	___x___	___x___
8. ☐	___x___	___x___	___x___	___x___	___x___
9. ☐	___x___	___x___	___x___	___x___	___x___
10. ☐	___x___	___x___	___x___	___x___	___x___
11. ☐	___x___	___x___	___x___	___x___	___x___
12. ☐	___x___	___x___	___x___	___x___	___x___

Workout Comments:

Supplements:

Sleep (hrs): 1 2 3 4 5 6 7 8 9 10+   Workout Rating: 1 2 3 4 5 6 7 8 9 10

Date:_____   Partner/Trainer:_____

Time:_____   Injuries:_____
start / finish

Location:_____   BP/RHR/WT:_____

☐ Warm-up ☐ Stretching ☐ Cool-down

Cardio / Class Phase

Focus:
☐ Fat Burn ☐ Random
☐ Interval ☐ Bootcamp
☐ Manual ☐ Circuit

Type	Duration (min)	HR (min/max)	Dist / Floors	Intensity	Calories

Training Phase

Focus:
☐ Upper: _____
☐ Lower: _____
☐ Full/Combo: _____

Exercise	Set 1 (WU) reps / weight	Set 2 reps / weight	Set 3 reps / weight	Set 4 reps / weight	Set 5 reps / weight
1.	___X___	___X___	___X___	___X___	___X___
2.	___X___	___X___	___X___	___X___	___X___
3.	___X___	___X___	___X___	___X___	___X___
4.	___X___	___X___	___X___	___X___	___X___
5.	___X___	___X___	___X___	___X___	___X___
6.	___X___	___X___	___X___	___X___	___X___
7.	___X___	___X___	___X___	___X___	___X___
8.	___X___	___X___	___X___	___X___	___X___
9.	___X___	___X___	___X___	___X___	___X___
10.	___X___	___X___	___X___	___X___	___X___
11.	___X___	___X___	___X___	___X___	___X___
12.	___X___	___X___	___X___	___X___	___X___

Workout Comments:

Supplements:

Sleep (hrs): 1 2 3 4 5 6 7 8 9 10+   Workout Rating: 1 2 3 4 5 6 7 8 9 10

Partner/Trainer:_____ Date:_____

Injuries:_____ Time:_____ start / finish

BP/RHR/WT:_____ Location:_____

☐ Warm-up ☐ Stretching ☐ Cool-down

Cardio / Class Phase

Focus:
☐ Fat Burn ☐ Random
☐ Interval ☐ Bootcamp
☐ Manual ☐ Circuit

Type	Duration (min)	HR (min/max)	Dist / Floors	Intensity	Calories

Training Phase

Focus:
☐ Upper: _____
☐ Lower: _____
☐ Full/Combo: _____

Exercise	Set 1 (WU) reps / weight	Set 2 reps / weight	Set 3 reps / weight	Set 4 reps / weight	Set 5 reps / weight
1. ☐	___ X ___	___ X ___	___ X ___	___ X ___	___ X ___
2. ☐	___ X ___	___ X ___	___ X ___	___ X ___	___ X ___
3. ☐	___ X ___	___ X ___	___ X ___	___ X ___	___ X ___
4. ☐	___ X ___	___ X ___	___ X ___	___ X ___	___ X ___
5. ☐	___ X ___	___ X ___	___ X ___	___ X ___	___ X ___
6. ☐	___ X ___	___ X ___	___ X ___	___ X ___	___ X ___
7. ☐	___ X ___	___ X ___	___ X ___	___ X ___	___ X ___
8. ☐	___ X ___	___ X ___	___ X ___	___ X ___	___ X ___
9. ☐	___ X ___	___ X ___	___ X ___	___ X ___	___ X ___
10. ☐	___ X ___	___ X ___	___ X ___	___ X ___	___ X ___
11. ☐	___ X ___	___ X ___	___ X ___	___ X ___	___ X ___
12. ☐	___ X ___	___ X ___	___ X ___	___ X ___	___ X ___

Workout Comments:

Supplements:

Sleep (hrs): 1 2 3 4 5 6 7 8 9 10+   Workout Rating: 1 2 3 4 5 6 7 8 9 10

Date:_____   Partner/Trainer:_____

Time:_____ start / finish _____   Injuries:_____

Location:_____   BP/RHR/WT:_____

☐ Warm-up   ☐ Stretching   ☐ Cool-down

Cardio / Class Phase

Focus:
☐ Fat Burn   ☐ Random
☐ Interval   ☐ Bootcamp
☐ Manual   ☐ Circuit

Type	Duration (min)	HR (min/max)	Dist / Floors	Intensity	Calories

Training Phase

Focus:
☐ Upper:_____
☐ Lower:_____
☐ Full/Combo:_____

Exercise	Set 1 (WU) reps / weight	Set 2 reps / weight	Set 3 reps / weight	Set 4 reps / weight	Set 5 reps / weight
1. ☐	___X___	___X___	___X___	___X___	___X___
2. ☐	___X___	___X___	___X___	___X___	___X___
3. ☐	___X___	___X___	___X___	___X___	___X___
4. ☐	___X___	___X___	___X___	___X___	___X___
5. ☐	___X___	___X___	___X___	___X___	___X___
6. ☐	___X___	___X___	___X___	___X___	___X___
7. ☐	___X___	___X___	___X___	___X___	___X___
8. ☐	___X___	___X___	___X___	___X___	___X___
9. ☐	___X___	___X___	___X___	___X___	___X___
10. ☐	___X___	___X___	___X___	___X___	___X___
11. ☐	___X___	___X___	___X___	___X___	___X___
12.	___X___	___X___	___X___	___X___	___X___

Workout Comments:

Supplements:

Sleep (hrs): 1 2 3 4 5 6 7 8 9 10+   Workout Rating: 1 2 3 4 5 6 7 8 9 10

Partner/Trainer:_____ Date:_____

Injuries:_____ Time:_____ start / finish

BP/RHR/WT:_____ Location:_____

☐ Warm-up ☐ Stretching ☐ Cool-down

Cardio / Class Phase

Focus:
☐ Fat Burn ☐ Random
☐ Interval ☐ Bootcamp
☐ Manual ☐ Circuit

Type	Duration (min)	HR (min/max)	Dist / Floors	Intensity	Calories

Training Phase

Focus:
☐ Upper: _____
☐ Lower: _____
☐ Full/Combo: _____

Exercise	Set 1 (WU) reps / weight	Set 2 reps / weight	Set 3 reps / weight	Set 4 reps / weight	Set 5 reps / weight
1.	___x___	___x___	___x___	___x___	___x___
2.	___x___	___x___	___x___	___x___	___x___
3.	___x___	___x___	___x___	___x___	___x___
4.	___x___	___x___	___x___	___x___	___x___
5.	___x___	___x___	___x___	___x___	___x___
6.	___x___	___x___	___x___	___x___	___x___
7.	___x___	___x___	___x___	___x___	___x___
8.	___x___	___x___	___x___	___x___	___x___
9.	___x___	___x___	___x___	___x___	___x___
10.	___x___	___x___	___x___	___x___	___x___
11.	___x___	___x___	___x___	___x___	___x___
12.	___x___	___x___	___x___	___x___	___x___

Workout Comments:

Supplements:

Sleep (hrs): 1 2 3 4 5 6 7 8 9 10+   Workout Rating: 1 2 3 4 5 6 7 8 9 10

Date:_____   Partner/Trainer:_____

Time:_____start / finish_____   Injuries:_____

Location:_____   BP/RHR/WT:_____

☐ Warm-up ☐ Stretching ☐ Cool-down

Cardio / Class Phase   Focus:

☐ Fat Burn ☐ Random
☐ Interval ☐ Bootcamp
☐ Manual   ☐ Circuit

Type	Duration (min)	HR (min/max)	Dist / Floors	Intensity	Calories

Training Phase   Focus:

☐ Upper: _____
☐ Lower: _____
☐ Full/Combo: _____

Exercise	Set 1 (WU) reps / weight	Set 2 reps / weight	Set 3 reps / weight	Set 4 reps / weight	Set 5 reps / weight
1. ☐	___X___	___X___	___X___	___X___	___X___
2. ☐	___X___	___X___	___X___	___X___	___X___
3. ☐	___X___	___X___	___X___	___X___	___X___
4. ☐	___X___	___X___	___X___	___X___	___X___
5. ☐	___X___	___X___	___X___	___X___	___X___
6. ☐	___X___	___X___	___X___	___X___	___X___
7. ☐	___X___	___X___	___X___	___X___	___X___
8. ☐	___X___	___X___	___X___	___X___	___X___
9. ☐	___X___	___X___	___X___	___X___	___X___
10. ☐	___X___	___X___	___X___	___X___	___X___
11. ☐	___X___	___X___	___X___	___X___	___X___
12. ☐	___X___	___X___	___X___	___X___	___X___

Workout Comments:

Supplements:

Sleep (hrs): 1 2 3 4 5 6 7 8 9 10+   Workout Rating: 1 2 3 4 5 6 7 8 9 10

Partner/Trainer:_____

Injuries:_____

BP/RHR/WT:_____

Date:_____

Time:_____ start / finish

Location:_____

☐ Warm-up ☐ Stretching ☐ Cool-down

Cardio / Class Phase

Focus:
☐ Fat Burn ☐ Random
☐ Interval ☐ Bootcamp
☐ Manual ☐ Circuit

Type	Duration (min)	HR (min/max)	Dist / Floors	Intensity	Calories

Training Phase

Focus:
☐ Upper: _____
☐ Lower: _____
☐ Full/Combo: _____

Exercise	Set 1 (WU) reps / weight	Set 2 reps / weight	Set 3 reps / weight	Set 4 reps / weight	Set 5 reps / weight
1.	___ X ___	___ X ___	___ X ___	___ X ___	___ X ___
2.	___ X ___	___ X ___	___ X ___	___ X ___	___ X ___
3.	___ X ___	___ X ___	___ X ___	___ X ___	___ X ___
4.	___ X ___	___ X ___	___ X ___	___ X ___	___ X ___
5.	___ X ___	___ X ___	___ X ___	___ X ___	___ X ___
6.	___ X ___	___ X ___	___ X ___	___ X ___	___ X ___
7.	___ X ___	___ X ___	___ X ___	___ X ___	___ X ___
8.	___ X ___	___ X ___	___ X ___	___ X ___	___ X ___
9.	___ X ___	___ X ___	___ X ___	___ X ___	___ X ___
10.	___ X ___	___ X ___	___ X ___	___ X ___	___ X ___
11.	___ X ___	___ X ___	___ X ___	___ X ___	___ X ___
12.	___ X ___	___ X ___	___ X ___	___ X ___	___ X ___

Workout Comments:

Supplements:

Sleep (hrs): 1 2 3 4 5 6 7 8 9 10+   **Workout Rating:** 1 2 3 4 5 6 7 8 9 10

Date:_____   Partner/Trainer:_____

Time:_____   Injuries:_____
          start / finish

Location:_____   BP/RHR/WT:_____

☐ Warm-up ☐ Stretching ☐ Cool-down

Cardio / Class Phase

Focus:
☐ Fat Burn ☐ Random
☐ Interval ☐ Bootcamp
☐ Manual ☐ Circuit

Type	Duration (min)	HR (min/max)	Dist / Floors	Intensity	Calories

Training Phase

Focus:
☐ Upper: _____
☐ Lower: _____
☐ Full/Combo: _____

Exercise	Set 1 (WU) reps / weight	Set 2 reps / weight	Set 3 reps / weight	Set 4 reps / weight	Set 5 reps / weight
1. ☐	___X___	___X___	___X___	___X___	___X___
2. ☐	___X___	___X___	___X___	___X___	___X___
3. ☐	___X___	___X___	___X___	___X___	___X___
4. ☐	___X___	___X___	___X___	___X___	___X___
5. ☐	___X___	___X___	___X___	___X___	___X___
6. ☐	___X___	___X___	___X___	___X___	___X___
7. ☐	___X___	___X___	___X___	___X___	___X___
8. ☐	___X___	___X___	___X___	___X___	___X___
9. ☐	___X___	___X___	___X___	___X___	___X___
10. ☐	___X___	___X___	___X___	___X___	___X___
11. ☐	___X___	___X___	___X___	___X___	___X___
12.	___X___	___X___	___X___	___X___	___X___

Workout Comments:

Supplements:

Sleep (hrs): 1 2 3 4 5 6 7 8 9 10+   Workout Rating: 1 2 3 4 5 6 7 8 9 10

Partner/Trainer:_____ Date:_____

Injuries:_____ Time:_____ start / finish

BP/RHR/WT:_____ Location:_____

☐ Warm-up ☐ Stretching ☐ Cool-down

Cardio / Class Phase   Focus:
☐ Fat Burn ☐ Random
☐ Interval ☐ Bootcamp
☐ Manual ☐ Circuit

Type	Duration (min)	HR (min/max)	Dist / Floors	Intensity	Calories

Training Phase   Focus:
☐ Upper: _____
☐ Lower: _____
☐ Full/Combo: _____

Exercise	Set 1 (WU) reps / weight	Set 2 reps / weight	Set 3 reps / weight	Set 4 reps / weight	Set 5 reps / weight
1.	__x__	__x__	__x__	__x__	__x__
2.	__x__	__x__	__x__	__x__	__x__
3.	__x__	__x__	__x__	__x__	__x__
4.	__x__	__x__	__x__	__x__	__x__
5.	__x__	__x__	__x__	__x__	__x__
6.	__x__	__x__	__x__	__x__	__x__
7.	__x__	__x__	__x__	__x__	__x__
8.	__x__	__x__	__x__	__x__	__x__
9.	__x__	__x__	__x__	__x__	__x__
10.	__x__	__x__	__x__	__x__	__x__
11.	__x__	__x__	__x__	__x__	__x__
12.	__x__	__x__	__x__	__x__	__x__

Workout Comments:

Supplements:

Sleep (hrs): 1 2 3 4 5 6 7 8 9 10+   Workout Rating: 1 2 3 4 5 6 7 8 9 10

Date:_____ Partner/Trainer:_____

Time:_____ start / finish Injuries:_____

Location:_____ BP/RHR/WT:_____

☐ Warm-up ☐ Stretching ☐ Cool-down

Cardio / Class Phase   **Focus:**

☐ Fat Burn ☐ Random
☐ Interval ☐ Bootcamp
☐ Manual ☐ Circuit

Type	Duration (min)	HR (min/max)	Dist / Floors	Intensity	Calories

Training Phase   **Focus:**

☐ Upper: _____
☐ Lower: _____
☐ Full/Combo: _____

Exercise	Set 1 (WU) reps / weight	Set 2 reps / weight	Set 3 reps / weight	Set 4 reps / weight	Set 5 reps / weight
1.	___X___	___X___	___X___	___X___	___X___
2.	___X___	___X___	___X___	___X___	___X___
3.	___X___	___X___	___X___	___X___	___X___
4.	___X___	___X___	___X___	___X___	___X___
5.	___X___	___X___	___X___	___X___	___X___
6.	___X___	___X___	___X___	___X___	___X___
7.	___X___	___X___	___X___	___X___	___X___
8.	___X___	___X___	___X___	___X___	___X___
9.	___X___	___X___	___X___	___X___	___X___
10.	___X___	___X___	___X___	___X___	___X___
11.	___X___	___X___	___X___	___X___	___X___
12.	___X___	___X___	___X___	___X___	___X___

Workout Comments:

Supplements:

Sleep (hrs): 1 2 3 4 5 6 7 8 9 10+   Workout Rating: 1 2 3 4 5 6 7 8 9 10

Partner/Trainer:_____

Injuries:_____

BP/RHR/WT:_____

Date:_____

Time:_____ start / finish

Location:_____

☐ Warm-up   ☐ Stretching   ☐ Cool-down

Cardio / Class Phase

Focus:
☐ Fat Burn   ☐ Random
☐ Interval   ☐ Bootcamp
☐ Manual   ☐ Circuit

Type	Duration (min)	HR (min/max)	Dist / Floors	Intensity	Calories

Training Phase

Focus:
☐ Upper: _____
☐ Lower: _____
☐ Full/Combo: _____

Exercise	Set 1 (WU) reps / weight	Set 2 reps / weight	Set 3 reps / weight	Set 4 reps / weight	Set 5 reps / weight
1.	___X___	___X___	___X___	___X___	___X___
2.	___X___	___X___	___X___	___X___	___X___
3.	___X___	___X___	___X___	___X___	___X___
4.	___X___	___X___	___X___	___X___	___X___
5.	___X___	___X___	___X___	___X___	___X___
6.	___X___	___X___	___X___	___X___	___X___
7.	___X___	___X___	___X___	___X___	___X___
8.	___X___	___X___	___X___	___X___	___X___
9.	___X___	___X___	___X___	___X___	___X___
10.	___X___	___X___	___X___	___X___	___X___
11.	___X___	___X___	___X___	___X___	___X___
12.	___X___	___X___	___X___	___X___	___X___

Workout Comments:

Supplements:

Sleep (hrs): 1 2 3 4 5 6 7 8 9 10+   Workout Rating: 1 2 3 4 5 6 7 8 9 10

Date:_____ Partner/Trainer:_____

Time:_____ start / finish _____ Injuries:_____

Location:_____ BP/RHR/WT:_____

☐ Warm-up ☐ Stretching ☐ Cool-down

Cardio / Class Phase   Focus:

☐ Fat Burn ☐ Random
☐ Interval ☐ Bootcamp
☐ Manual   ☐ Circuit

Type	Duration (min)	HR (min/max)	Dist / Floors	Intensity	Calories

Training Phase   Focus:

☐ Upper: _____
☐ Lower: _____
☐ Full/Combo: _____

Exercise	Set 1 (WU) reps / weight	Set 2 reps / weight	Set 3 reps / weight	Set 4 reps / weight	Set 5 reps / weight
1.	___X___	___X___	___X___	___X___	___X___
2.	___X___	___X___	___X___	___X___	___X___
3.	___X___	___X___	___X___	___X___	___X___
4.	___X___	___X___	___X___	___X___	___X___
5.	___X___	___X___	___X___	___X___	___X___
6.	___X___	___X___	___X___	___X___	___X___
7.	___X___	___X___	___X___	___X___	___X___
8.	___X___	___X___	___X___	___X___	___X___
9.	___X___	___X___	___X___	___X___	___X___
10.	___X___	___X___	___X___	___X___	___X___
11.	___X___	___X___	___X___	___X___	___X___
12.	___X___	___X___	___X___	___X___	___X___

Workout Comments:

Supplements:

Sleep (hrs): 1 2 3 4 5 6 7 8 9 10+   Workout Rating: 1 2 3 4 5 6 7 8 9 10

Partner/Trainer:_____ Date:_____

Injuries:_____ Time:_____ start / finish ___

BP/RHR/WT:_____ Location:_____

☐ Warm-up ☐ Stretching ☐ Cool-down

Cardio / Class Phase

Focus:
☐ Fat Burn ☐ Random
☐ Interval ☐ Bootcamp
☐ Manual ☐ Circuit

Type	Duration (min)	HR (min/max)	Dist / Floors	Intensity	Calories

Training Phase

Focus:
☐ Upper: _____
☐ Lower: _____
☐ Full/Combo: _____

Exercise	Set 1 (WU) reps / weight	Set 2 reps / weight	Set 3 reps / weight	Set 4 reps / weight	Set 5 reps / weight
1. ☐	___ X ___	___ X ___	___ X ___	___ X ___	___ X ___
2. ☐	___ X ___	___ X ___	___ X ___	___ X ___	___ X ___
3. ☐	___ X ___	___ X ___	___ X ___	___ X ___	___ X ___
4. ☐	___ X ___	___ X ___	___ X ___	___ X ___	___ X ___
5. ☐	___ X ___	___ X ___	___ X ___	___ X ___	___ X ___
6. ☐	___ X ___	___ X ___	___ X ___	___ X ___	___ X ___
7. ☐	___ X ___	___ X ___	___ X ___	___ X ___	___ X ___
8. ☐	___ X ___	___ X ___	___ X ___	___ X ___	___ X ___
9. ☐	___ X ___	___ X ___	___ X ___	___ X ___	___ X ___
10. ☐	___ X ___	___ X ___	___ X ___	___ X ___	___ X ___
11. ☐	___ X ___	___ X ___	___ X ___	___ X ___	___ X ___
12.	___ X ___	___ X ___	___ X ___	___ X ___	___ X ___

Workout Comments:

Supplements:

Sleep (hrs): 1 2 3 4 5 6 7 8 9 10+   Workout Rating: 1 2 3 4 5 6 7 8 9 10

Date:_____   Partner/Trainer:_____

Time:_____   Injuries:_____
       start / finish

Location:_____   BP/RHR/WT:_____

☐ Warm-up ☐ Stretching ☐ Cool-down

Cardio / Class Phase

Focus:
☐ Fat Burn ☐ Random
☐ Interval ☐ Bootcamp
☐ Manual   ☐ Circuit

Type	Duration (min)	HR (min/max)	Dist / Floors	Intensity	Calories

Training Phase

Focus:
☐ Upper: _____
☐ Lower: _____
☐ Full/Combo: _____

Exercise	Set 1 (WU) reps / weight	Set 2 reps / weight	Set 3 reps / weight	Set 4 reps / weight	Set 5 reps / weight
1. ☐	___ X ___	___ X ___	___ X ___	___ X ___	___ X ___
2. ☐	___ X ___	___ X ___	___ X ___	___ X ___	___ X ___
3. ☐	___ X ___	___ X ___	___ X ___	___ X ___	___ X ___
4. ☐	___ X ___	___ X ___	___ X ___	___ X ___	___ X ___
5. ☐	___ X ___	___ X ___	___ X ___	___ X ___	___ X ___
6. ☐	___ X ___	___ X ___	___ X ___	___ X ___	___ X ___
7. ☐	___ X ___	___ X ___	___ X ___	___ X ___	___ X ___
8. ☐	___ X ___	___ X ___	___ X ___	___ X ___	___ X ___
9. ☐	___ X ___	___ X ___	___ X ___	___ X ___	___ X ___
10. ☐	___ X ___	___ X ___	___ X ___	___ X ___	___ X ___
11. ☐	___ X ___	___ X ___	___ X ___	___ X ___	___ X ___
12.	___ X ___	___ X ___	___ X ___	___ X ___	___ X ___

Workout Comments:

Supplements:

Sleep (hrs): 1 2 3 4 5 6 7 8 9 10+   Workout Rating: 1 2 3 4 5 6 7 8 9 10

Partner/Trainer:_____   Date:_____

Injuries:_____   Time:_____ start / finish

BP/RHR/WT:_____   Location:_____

☐ Warm-up ☐ Stretching ☐ Cool-down

Cardio / Class Phase Focus:

☐ Fat Burn ☐ Random
☐ Interval ☐ Bootcamp
☐ Manual ☐ Circuit

Type	Duration (min)	HR (min/max)	Dist / Floors	Intensity	Calories

Training Phase Focus:

☐ Upper: _____
☐ Lower: _____
☐ Full/Combo: _____

Exercise	Set 1 (WU) reps / weight	Set 2 reps / weight	Set 3 reps / weight	Set 4 reps / weight	Set 5 reps / weight
1. ☐	___x___	___x___	___x___	___x___	___x___
2. ☐	___x___	___x___	___x___	___x___	___x___
3. ☐	___x___	___x___	___x___	___x___	___x___
4. ☐	___x___	___x___	___x___	___x___	___x___
5. ☐	___x___	___x___	___x___	___x___	___x___
6. ☐	___x___	___x___	___x___	___x___	___x___
7. ☐	___x___	___x___	___x___	___x___	___x___
8. ☐	___x___	___x___	___x___	___x___	___x___
9. ☐	___x___	___x___	___x___	___x___	___x___
10. ☐	___x___	___x___	___x___	___x___	___x___
11. ☐	___x___	___x___	___x___	___x___	___x___
12. ☐	___x___	___x___	___x___	___x___	___x___

Workout Comments:

Supplements:

Sleep (hrs): 1 2 3 4 5 6 7 8 9 10+   Workout Rating: 1 2 3 4 5 6 7 8 9 10

Date:_____   Partner/Trainer:_____
Time:_____ start / finish _____   Injuries:_____
Location:_____   BP/RHR/WT:_____

☐ Warm-up ☐ Stretching ☐ Cool-down

Cardio / Class Phase   Focus:

☐ Fat Burn ☐ Random
☐ Interval ☐ Bootcamp
☐ Manual   ☐ Circuit

Type	Duration (min)	HR (min/max)	Dist / Floors	Intensity	Calories

Training Phase   Focus:

☐ Upper: _____
☐ Lower: _____
☐ Full/Combo: _____

Exercise	Set 1 (WU) reps / weight	Set 2 reps / weight	Set 3 reps / weight	Set 4 reps / weight	Set 5 reps / weight
1.	___X___	___X___	___X___	___X___	___X___
2.	___X___	___X___	___X___	___X___	___X___
3.	___X___	___X___	___X___	___X___	___X___
4.	___X___	___X___	___X___	___X___	___X___
5.	___X___	___X___	___X___	___X___	___X___
6.	___X___	___X___	___X___	___X___	___X___
7.	___X___	___X___	___X___	___X___	___X___
8.	___X___	___X___	___X___	___X___	___X___
9.	___X___	___X___	___X___	___X___	___X___
10.	___X___	___X___	___X___	___X___	___X___
11.	___X___	___X___	___X___	___X___	___X___
12.	___X___	___X___	___X___	___X___	___X___

Workout Comments:

Supplements:

Sleep (hrs): 1 2 3 4 5 6 7 8 9 10+   Workout Rating: 1 2 3 4 5 6 7 8 9 10

Partner/Trainer:_____

Injuries:_____

BP/RHR/WT:_____

Date:_____

Time:_____ start / finish

Location:_____

☐ Warm-up   ☐ Stretching   ☐ Cool-down

Cardio / Class Phase

Focus:
☐ Fat Burn   ☐ Random
☐ Interval   ☐ Bootcamp
☐ Manual   ☐ Circuit

Type	Duration (min)	HR (min/max)	Dist / Floors	Intensity	Calories

Training Phase

Focus:
☐ Upper: _____
☐ Lower: _____
☐ Full/Combo: _____

Exercise	Set 1 (WU) reps / weight	Set 2 reps / weight	Set 3 reps / weight	Set 4 reps / weight	Set 5 reps / weight
1.	X	X	X	X	X
2.	X	X	X	X	X
3.	X	X	X	X	X
4.	X	X	X	X	X
5.	X	X	X	X	X
6.	X	X	X	X	X
7.	X	X	X	X	X
8.	X	X	X	X	X
9.	X	X	X	X	X
10.	X	X	X	X	X
11.	X	X	X	X	X
12.	X	X	X	X	X

Workout Comments:

Supplements:

Sleep (hrs): 1 2 3 4 5 6 7 8 9 10+   **Workout Rating:** 1 2 3 4 5 6 7 8 9 10

Date:_____   Partner/Trainer:_____

Time:_____ start / finish   Injuries:_____

Location:_____   BP/RHR/WT:_____

☐ Warm-up   ☐ Stretching   ☐ Cool-down

Cardio / Class Phase

Focus:
☐ Fat Burn   ☐ Random
☐ Interval   ☐ Bootcamp
☐ Manual   ☐ Circuit

Type	Duration (min)	HR (min/max)	Dist / Floors	Intensity	Calories

Training Phase   **Focus:**

☐ Upper: _____
☐ Lower: _____
☐ Full/Combo: _____

Exercise	Set 1 (WU) reps / weight	Set 2 reps / weight	Set 3 reps / weight	Set 4 reps / weight	Set 5 reps / weight
1.	___X___	___X___	___X___	___X___	___X___
2.	___X___	___X___	___X___	___X___	___X___
3.	___X___	___X___	___X___	___X___	___X___
4.	___X___	___X___	___X___	___X___	___X___
5.	___X___	___X___	___X___	___X___	___X___
6.	___X___	___X___	___X___	___X___	___X___
7.	___X___	___X___	___X___	___X___	___X___
8.	___X___	___X___	___X___	___X___	___X___
9.	___X___	___X___	___X___	___X___	___X___
10.	___X___	___X___	___X___	___X___	___X___
11.	___X___	___X___	___X___	___X___	___X___
12.	___X___	___X___	___X___	___X___	___X___

Workout Comments:

Supplements:

Sleep (hrs): 1 2 3 4 5 6 7 8 9 10+   Workout Rating: 1 2 3 4 5 6 7 8 9 10

Partner/Trainer:_____ Date:_____

Injuries:_____ Time:_____ start / finish _____

BP/RHR/WT:_____ Location:_____

☐ Warm-up ☐ Stretching ☐ Cool-down

Cardio / Class Phase Focus:

☐ Fat Burn ☐ Random
☐ Interval ☐ Bootcamp
☐ Manual ☐ Circuit

Type	Duration (min)	HR (min/max)	Dist / Floors	Intensity	Calories

Training Phase Focus:

☐ Upper: _____
☐ Lower: _____
☐ Full/Combo: _____

Exercise	Set 1 (WU) reps / weight	Set 2 reps / weight	Set 3 reps / weight	Set 4 reps / weight	Set 5 reps / weight
1.	___X___	___X___	___X___	___X___	___X___
2.	___X___	___X___	___X___	___X___	___X___
3.	___X___	___X___	___X___	___X___	___X___
4.	___X___	___X___	___X___	___X___	___X___
5.	___X___	___X___	___X___	___X___	___X___
6.	___X___	___X___	___X___	___X___	___X___
7.	___X___	___X___	___X___	___X___	___X___
8.	___X___	___X___	___X___	___X___	___X___
9.	___X___	___X___	___X___	___X___	___X___
10.	___X___	___X___	___X___	___X___	___X___
11.	___X___	___X___	___X___	___X___	___X___
12.	___X___	___X___	___X___	___X___	___X___

Workout Comments:

Supplements:

Sleep (hrs): 1 2 3 4 5 6 7 8 9 10+   Workout Rating: 1 2 3 4 5 6 7 8 9 10

Date:_____ Partner/Trainer:_____

Time:_____ Injuries:_____
         start / finish

Location:_____ BP/RHR/WT:_____

☐ Warm-up ☐ Stretching ☐ Cool-down

Cardio / Class Phase   Focus:

☐ Fat Burn ☐ Random
☐ Interval ☐ Bootcamp
☐ Manual ☐ Circuit

Type	Duration (min)	HR (min/max)	Dist / Floors	Intensity	Calories

Training Phase   Focus:

☐ Upper: _____
☐ Lower: _____
☐ Full/Combo: _____

Exercise	Set 1 (WU) reps / weight	Set 2 reps / weight	Set 3 reps / weight	Set 4 reps / weight	Set 5 reps / weight
1. ☐	___X___	___X___	___X___	___X___	___X___
2. ☐	___X___	___X___	___X___	___X___	___X___
3. ☐	___X___	___X___	___X___	___X___	___X___
4. ☐	___X___	___X___	___X___	___X___	___X___
5. ☐	___X___	___X___	___X___	___X___	___X___
6. ☐	___X___	___X___	___X___	___X___	___X___
7. ☐	___X___	___X___	___X___	___X___	___X___
8. ☐	___X___	___X___	___X___	___X___	___X___
9. ☐	___X___	___X___	___X___	___X___	___X___
10. ☐	___X___	___X___	___X___	___X___	___X___
11. ☐	___X___	___X___	___X___	___X___	___X___
12. ☐	___X___	___X___	___X___	___X___	___X___

Workout Comments:

Supplements:

Sleep (hrs): 1 2 3 4 5 6 7 8 9 10+   Workout Rating: 1 2 3 4 5 6 7 8 9 10

Partner/Trainer:_____ Date:_____

Injuries:_____ Time:_____ start / finish

BP/RHR/WT:_____ Location:_____

☐ Warm-up ☐ Stretching ☐ Cool-down

Cardio / Class Phase   Focus:

☐ Fat Burn ☐ Random
☐ Interval ☐ Bootcamp
☐ Manual ☐ Circuit

Type	Duration (min)	HR (min/max)	Dist / Floors	Intensity	Calories

Training Phase   Focus:

☐ Upper: _____
☐ Lower: _____
☐ Full/Combo: _____

Exercise	Set 1 (WU) reps / weight	Set 2 reps / weight	Set 3 reps / weight	Set 4 reps / weight	Set 5 reps / weight
1.	___X___	___X___	___X___	___X___	___X___
2.	___X___	___X___	___X___	___X___	___X___
3.	___X___	___X___	___X___	___X___	___X___
4.	___X___	___X___	___X___	___X___	___X___
5.	___X___	___X___	___X___	___X___	___X___
6.	___X___	___X___	___X___	___X___	___X___
7.	___X___	___X___	___X___	___X___	___X___
8.	___X___	___X___	___X___	___X___	___X___
9.	___X___	___X___	___X___	___X___	___X___
10.	___X___	___X___	___X___	___X___	___X___
11.	___X___	___X___	___X___	___X___	___X___
12.	___X___	___X___	___X___	___X___	___X___

Workout Comments:

Supplements:

Sleep (hrs): 1 2 3 4 5 6 7 8 9 10+   Workout Rating: 1 2 3 4 5 6 7 8 9 10

Date:_____ Partner/Trainer:_____

Time:_____ start / finish _____ Injuries:_____

Location:_____ BP/RHR/WT:_____

☐ Warm-up ☐ Stretching ☐ Cool-down

Cardio / Class Phase

Focus:
☐ Fat Burn ☐ Random
☐ Interval ☐ Bootcamp
☐ Manual ☐ Circuit

Type	Duration (min)	HR (min/max)	Dist / Floors	Intensity	Calories

Training Phase

Focus:
☐ Upper: _____
☐ Lower: _____
☐ Full/Combo: _____

Exercise	Set 1 (WU) reps / weight	Set 2 reps / weight	Set 3 reps / weight	Set 4 reps / weight	Set 5 reps / weight
1.	___X___	___X___	___X___	___X___	___X___
2.	___X___	___X___	___X___	___X___	___X___
3.	___X___	___X___	___X___	___X___	___X___
4.	___X___	___X___	___X___	___X___	___X___
5.	___X___	___X___	___X___	___X___	___X___
6.	___X___	___X___	___X___	___X___	___X___
7.	___X___	___X___	___X___	___X___	___X___
8.	___X___	___X___	___X___	___X___	___X___
9.	___X___	___X___	___X___	___X___	___X___
10.	___X___	___X___	___X___	___X___	___X___
11.	___X___	___X___	___X___	___X___	___X___
12.	___X___	___X___	___X___	___X___	___X___

Workout Comments:

Supplements:

Sleep (hrs): 1 2 3 4 5 6 7 8 9 10+   Workout Rating: 1 2 3 4 5 6 7 8 9 10

Partner/Trainer:_____ Date:_____

Injuries:_____ Time:_____ start / finish

BP/RHR/WT:_____ Location:_____

☐ Warm-up ☐ Stretching ☐ Cool-down

Cardio / Class Phase

Focus:
☐ Fat Burn ☐ Random
☐ Interval ☐ Bootcamp
☐ Manual ☐ Circuit

Type	Duration (min)	HR (min/max)	Dist / Floors	Intensity	Calories

Training Phase

Focus:
☐ Upper: _____
☐ Lower: _____
☐ Full/Combo: _____

Exercise	Set 1 (WU) reps / weight	Set 2 reps / weight	Set 3 reps / weight	Set 4 reps / weight	Set 5 reps / weight
1.	___X___	___X___	___X___	___X___	___X___
2.	___X___	___X___	___X___	___X___	___X___
3.	___X___	___X___	___X___	___X___	___X___
4.	___X___	___X___	___X___	___X___	___X___
5.	___X___	___X___	___X___	___X___	___X___
6.	___X___	___X___	___X___	___X___	___X___
7.	___X___	___X___	___X___	___X___	___X___
8.	___X___	___X___	___X___	___X___	___X___
9.	___X___	___X___	___X___	___X___	___X___
10.	___X___	___X___	___X___	___X___	___X___
11.	___X___	___X___	___X___	___X___	___X___
12.	___X___	___X___	___X___	___X___	___X___

Workout Comments:

Supplements:

Sleep (hrs): 1 2 3 4 5 6 7 8 9 10+   Workout Rating: 1 2 3 4 5 6 7 8 9 10

Date:_____   Partner/Trainer:_____

Time:_____ start / finish _____   Injuries:_____

Location:_____   BP/RHR/WT:_____

☐ Warm-up ☐ Stretching ☐ Cool-down

Cardio / Class Phase **Focus**:

☐ Fat Burn ☐ Random
☐ Interval ☐ Bootcamp
☐ Manual   ☐ Circuit

Type	Duration (min)	HR (min/max)	Dist / Floors	Intensity	Calories

Training Phase **Focus**:

☐ Upper: _____
☐ Lower: _____
☐ Full/Combo: _____

Exercise	Set 1 (WU) reps / weight	Set 2 reps / weight	Set 3 reps / weight	Set 4 reps / weight	Set 5 reps / weight
1.	___X___	___X___	___X___	___X___	___X___
2.	___X___	___X___	___X___	___X___	___X___
3.	___X___	___X___	___X___	___X___	___X___
4.	___X___	___X___	___X___	___X___	___X___
5.	___X___	___X___	___X___	___X___	___X___
6.	___X___	___X___	___X___	___X___	___X___
7.	___X___	___X___	___X___	___X___	___X___
8.	___X___	___X___	___X___	___X___	___X___
9.	___X___	___X___	___X___	___X___	___X___
10.	___X___	___X___	___X___	___X___	___X___
11.	___X___	___X___	___X___	___X___	___X___
12.	___X___	___X___	___X___	___X___	___X___

Workout Comments:

Supplements:

Sleep (hrs): 1 2 3 4 5 6 7 8 9 10+   Workout Rating: 1 2 3 4 5 6 7 8 9 10

Partner/Trainer:_____ Date:_____

Injuries:_____ Time:_____ start / finish

BP/RHR/WT:_____ Location:_____

☐ Warm-up ☐ Stretching ☐ Cool-down

Cardio / Class Phase

Focus:
☐ Fat Burn ☐ Random
☐ Interval ☐ Bootcamp
☐ Manual ☐ Circuit

Type	Duration (min)	HR (min/max)	Dist / Floors	Intensity	Calories

Training Phase

Focus:
☐ Upper: _____
☐ Lower: _____
☐ Full/Combo: _____

Exercise	Set 1 (WU) reps / weight	Set 2 reps / weight	Set 3 reps / weight	Set 4 reps / weight	Set 5 reps / weight
1.	___X___	___X___	___X___	___X___	___X___
2.	___X___	___X___	___X___	___X___	___X___
3.	___X___	___X___	___X___	___X___	___X___
4.	___X___	___X___	___X___	___X___	___X___
5.	___X___	___X___	___X___	___X___	___X___
6.	___X___	___X___	___X___	___X___	___X___
7.	___X___	___X___	___X___	___X___	___X___
8.	___X___	___X___	___X___	___X___	___X___
9.	___X___	___X___	___X___	___X___	___X___
10.	___X___	___X___	___X___	___X___	___X___
11.	___X___	___X___	___X___	___X___	___X___
12.	___X___	___X___	___X___	___X___	___X___

Workout Comments:

Supplements:

Sleep (hrs): 1 2 3 4 5 6 7 8 9 10+   Workout Rating: 1 2 3 4 5 6 7 8 9 10

Date:_____   Partner/Trainer:_____

Time:_____ start / finish   Injuries:_____

Location:_____   BP/RHR/WT:_____

☐ Warm-up ☐ Stretching ☐ Cool-down

Cardio / Class Phase Focus:

☐ Fat Burn ☐ Random
☐ Interval ☐ Bootcamp
☐ Manual ☐ Circuit

Type	Duration (min)	HR (min/max)	Dist / Floors	Intensity	Calories

Training Phase Focus:

☐ Upper: _____
☐ Lower: _____
☐ Full/Combo: _____

Exercise	Set 1 (WU) reps / weight	Set 2 reps / weight	Set 3 reps / weight	Set 4 reps / weight	Set 5 reps / weight
1.	___ x ___	___ x ___	___ x ___	___ x ___	___ x ___
2.	___ x ___	___ x ___	___ x ___	___ x ___	___ x ___
3.	___ x ___	___ x ___	___ x ___	___ x ___	___ x ___
4.	___ x ___	___ x ___	___ x ___	___ x ___	___ x ___
5.	___ x ___	___ x ___	___ x ___	___ x ___	___ x ___
6.	___ x ___	___ x ___	___ x ___	___ x ___	___ x ___
7.	___ x ___	___ x ___	___ x ___	___ x ___	___ x ___
8.	___ x ___	___ x ___	___ x ___	___ x ___	___ x ___
9.	___ x ___	___ x ___	___ x ___	___ x ___	___ x ___
10.	___ x ___	___ x ___	___ x ___	___ x ___	___ x ___
11.	___ x ___	___ x ___	___ x ___	___ x ___	___ x ___
12.	___ x ___	___ x ___	___ x ___	___ x ___	___ x ___

Workout Comments:

Supplements:

Sleep (hrs): 1 2 3 4 5 6 7 8 9 10+   Workout Rating: 1 2 3 4 5 6 7 8 9 10

Partner/Trainer:_____ Date:_____

Injuries:_____ Time:_____ start / finish

BP/RHR/WT:_____ Location:_____

☐ Warm-up ☐ Stretching ☐ Cool-down

Cardio / Class Phase Focus:

☐ Fat Burn ☐ Random
☐ Interval ☐ Bootcamp
☐ Manual ☐ Circuit

Type	Duration (min)	HR (min/max)	Dist / Floors	Intensity	Calories

Training Phase Focus:

☐ Upper: _____
☐ Lower: _____
☐ Full/Combo: _____

Exercise	Set 1 (WU) reps / weight	Set 2 reps / weight	Set 3 reps / weight	Set 4 reps / weight	Set 5 reps / weight
1.	___x___	___x___	___x___	___x___	___x___
2.	___x___	___x___	___x___	___x___	___x___
3.	___x___	___x___	___x___	___x___	___x___
4.	___x___	___x___	___x___	___x___	___x___
5.	___x___	___x___	___x___	___x___	___x___
6.	___x___	___x___	___x___	___x___	___x___
7.	___x___	___x___	___x___	___x___	___x___
8.	___x___	___x___	___x___	___x___	___x___
9.	___x___	___x___	___x___	___x___	___x___
10.	___x___	___x___	___x___	___x___	___x___
11.	___x___	___x___	___x___	___x___	___x___
12.	___x___	___x___	___x___	___x___	___x___

Workout Comments:

Supplements:

Sleep (hrs): 1 2 3 4 5 6 7 8 9 10+   Workout Rating: 1 2 3 4 5 6 7 8 9 10

Date:_____ Partner/Trainer:_____

Time:_____ start / finish Injuries:_____

Location:_____ BP/RHR/WT:_____

☐ Warm-up ☐ Stretching ☐ Cool-down

Cardio / Class Phase Focus:

☐ Fat Burn ☐ Random
☐ Interval ☐ Bootcamp
☐ Manual ☐ Circuit

Type	Duration (min)	HR (min/max)	Dist / Floors	Intensity	Calories

Training Phase Focus:

☐ Upper: _____
☐ Lower: _____
☐ Full/Combo: _____

Exercise	Set 1 (WU) reps / weight	Set 2 reps / weight	Set 3 reps / weight	Set 4 reps / weight	Set 5 reps / weight
1.	___X___	___X___	___X___	___X___	___X___
2.	___X___	___X___	___X___	___X___	___X___
3.	___X___	___X___	___X___	___X___	___X___
4.	___X___	___X___	___X___	___X___	___X___
5.	___X___	___X___	___X___	___X___	___X___
6.	___X___	___X___	___X___	___X___	___X___
7.	___X___	___X___	___X___	___X___	___X___
8.	___X___	___X___	___X___	___X___	___X___
9.	___X___	___X___	___X___	___X___	___X___
10.	___X___	___X___	___X___	___X___	___X___
11.	___X___	___X___	___X___	___X___	___X___
12.	___X___	___X___	___X___	___X___	___X___

Workout Comments:

Supplements:

Sleep (hrs): 1 2 3 4 5 6 7 8 9 10+   Workout Rating: 1 2 3 4 5 6 7 8 9 10

Partner/Trainer:_____   Date:_____

Injuries:_____   Time:_____ start / finish _____

BP/RHR/WT:_____   Location:_____

☐ Warm-up   ☐ Stretching   ☐ Cool-down

Cardio / Class Phase   Focus:

☐ Fat Burn   ☐ Random
☐ Interval   ☐ Bootcamp
☐ Manual   ☐ Circuit

Type	Duration (min)	HR (min/max)	Dist / Floors	Intensity	Calories

Training Phase   Focus:

☐ Upper: _____
☐ Lower: _____
☐ Full/Combo: _____

Exercise	Set 1 (WU) reps / weight	Set 2 reps / weight	Set 3 reps / weight	Set 4 reps / weight	Set 5 reps / weight
1.	___x___	___x___	___x___	___x___	___x___
2.	___x___	___x___	___x___	___x___	___x___
3.	___x___	___x___	___x___	___x___	___x___
4.	___x___	___x___	___x___	___x___	___x___
5.	___x___	___x___	___x___	___x___	___x___
6.	___x___	___x___	___x___	___x___	___x___
7.	___x___	___x___	___x___	___x___	___x___
8.	___x___	___x___	___x___	___x___	___x___
9.	___x___	___x___	___x___	___x___	___x___
10.	___x___	___x___	___x___	___x___	___x___
11.	___x___	___x___	___x___	___x___	___x___
12.	___x___	___x___	___x___	___x___	___x___

Workout Comments:

Supplements:

Sleep (hrs): 1 2 3 4 5 6 7 8 9 10+   Workout Rating: 1 2 3 4 5 6 7 8 9 10

Date:_____   Partner/Trainer:_____

Time:_____ start / finish   Injuries:_____

Location:_____   BP/RHR/WT:_____

☐ Warm-up ☐ Stretching ☐ Cool-down

Cardio / Class Phase

Focus:
☐ Fat Burn ☐ Random
☐ Interval ☐ Bootcamp
☐ Manual ☐ Circuit

Type	Duration (min)	HR (min/max)	Dist / Floors	Intensity	Calories

Training Phase

Focus:
☐ Upper: _____
☐ Lower: _____
☐ Full/Combo: _____

Exercise	Set 1 (WU) reps / weight	Set 2 reps / weight	Set 3 reps / weight	Set 4 reps / weight	Set 5 reps / weight
1.	___ X ___	___ X ___	___ X ___	___ X ___	___ X ___
2.	___ X ___	___ X ___	___ X ___	___ X ___	___ X ___
3.	___ X ___	___ X ___	___ X ___	___ X ___	___ X ___
4.	___ X ___	___ X ___	___ X ___	___ X ___	___ X ___
5.	___ X ___	___ X ___	___ X ___	___ X ___	___ X ___
6.	___ X ___	___ X ___	___ X ___	___ X ___	___ X ___
7.	___ X ___	___ X ___	___ X ___	___ X ___	___ X ___
8.	___ X ___	___ X ___	___ X ___	___ X ___	___ X ___
9.	___ X ___	___ X ___	___ X ___	___ X ___	___ X ___
10.	___ X ___	___ X ___	___ X ___	___ X ___	___ X ___
11.	___ X ___	___ X ___	___ X ___	___ X ___	___ X ___
12.	___ X ___	___ X ___	___ X ___	___ X ___	___ X ___

Workout Comments:

Supplements:

Sleep (hrs): 1 2 3 4 5 6 7 8 9 10+   Workout Rating: 1 2 3 4 5 6 7 8 9 10

Partner/Trainer:_____ Date:_____

Injuries:_____ Time:_____ start / finish _____

BP/RHR/WT:_____ Location:_____

☐ Warm-up ☐ Stretching ☐ Cool-down

Cardio / Class Phase   Focus:

☐ Fat Burn ☐ Random
☐ Interval ☐ Bootcamp
☐ Manual ☐ Circuit

Type	Duration (min)	HR (min/max)	Dist / Floors	Intensity	Calories

Training Phase   Focus:

☐ Upper: _____
☐ Lower: _____
☐ Full/Combo: _____

Exercise	Set 1 (WU) reps / weight	Set 2 reps / weight	Set 3 reps / weight	Set 4 reps / weight	Set 5 reps / weight
1.	___x___	___x___	___x___	___x___	___x___
2.	___x___	___x___	___x___	___x___	___x___
3.	___x___	___x___	___x___	___x___	___x___
4.	___x___	___x___	___x___	___x___	___x___
5.	___x___	___x___	___x___	___x___	___x___
6.	___x___	___x___	___x___	___x___	___x___
7.	___x___	___x___	___x___	___x___	___x___
8.	___x___	___x___	___x___	___x___	___x___
9.	___x___	___x___	___x___	___x___	___x___
10.	___x___	___x___	___x___	___x___	___x___
11.	___x___	___x___	___x___	___x___	___x___
12.	___x___	___x___	___x___	___x___	___x___

Workout Comments:

Supplements:

Sleep (hrs): 1 2 3 4 5 6 7 8 9 10+   Workout Rating: 1 2 3 4 5 6 7 8 9 10

Date:_____   Partner/Trainer:_____

Time:_____   Injuries:_____
      start / finish

Location:_____   BP/RHR/WT:_____

☐ Warm-up ☐ Stretching ☐ Cool-down

Cardio / Class Phase   Focus:

☐ Fat Burn   ☐ Random
☐ Interval   ☐ Bootcamp
☐ Manual   ☐ Circuit

Type	Duration (min)	HR (min/max)	Dist / Floors	Intensity	Calories

Training Phase   Focus:

☐ Upper: _____
☐ Lower: _____
☐ Full/Combo: _____

Exercise	Set 1 (WU) reps / weight	Set 2 reps / weight	Set 3 reps / weight	Set 4 reps / weight	Set 5 reps / weight
1. ☐	___X___	___X___	___X___	___X___	___X___
2. ☐	___X___	___X___	___X___	___X___	___X___
3. ☐	___X___	___X___	___X___	___X___	___X___
4. ☐	___X___	___X___	___X___	___X___	___X___
5. ☐	___X___	___X___	___X___	___X___	___X___
6. ☐	___X___	___X___	___X___	___X___	___X___
7. ☐	___X___	___X___	___X___	___X___	___X___
8. ☐	___X___	___X___	___X___	___X___	___X___
9. ☐	___X___	___X___	___X___	___X___	___X___
10. ☐	___X___	___X___	___X___	___X___	___X___
11. ☐	___X___	___X___	___X___	___X___	___X___
12.	___X___	___X___	___X___	___X___	___X___

Workout Comments:

Supplements:

Sleep (hrs): 1 2 3 4 5 6 7 8 9 10+   Workout Rating: 1 2 3 4 5 6 7 8 9 10

Partner/Trainer:_____ Date:_____

Injuries:_____ Time:_____ start / finish _____

BP/RHR/WT:_____ Location:_____

☐ Warm-up ☐ Stretching ☐ Cool-down

Cardio / Class Phase

Focus:
☐ Fat Burn ☐ Random
☐ Interval ☐ Bootcamp
☐ Manual ☐ Circuit

Type	Duration (min)	HR (min/max)	Dist / Floors	Intensity	Calories

Training Phase

Focus:
☐ Upper: _____
☐ Lower: _____
☐ Full/Combo: _____

Exercise	Set 1 (WU) reps / weight	Set 2 reps / weight	Set 3 reps / weight	Set 4 reps / weight	Set 5 reps / weight
1.	___x___	___x___	___x___	___x___	___x___
2.	___x___	___x___	___x___	___x___	___x___
3.	___x___	___x___	___x___	___x___	___x___
4.	___x___	___x___	___x___	___x___	___x___
5.	___x___	___x___	___x___	___x___	___x___
6.	___x___	___x___	___x___	___x___	___x___
7.	___x___	___x___	___x___	___x___	___x___
8.	___x___	___x___	___x___	___x___	___x___
9.	___x___	___x___	___x___	___x___	___x___
10.	___x___	___x___	___x___	___x___	___x___
11.	___x___	___x___	___x___	___x___	___x___
12.	___x___	___x___	___x___	___x___	___x___

Workout Comments:

Supplements:

Sleep (hrs): 1 2 3 4 5 6 7 8 9 10+   Workout Rating: 1 2 3 4 5 6 7 8 9 10

Date:_____	Partner/Trainer:_____
Time:_____ start / finish _____	Injuries:_____
Location:_____	BP/RHR/WT:_____

☐ Warm-up ☐ Stretching ☐ Cool-down

Cardio / Class Phase   Focus:

☐ Fat Burn ☐ Random
☐ Interval ☐ Bootcamp
☐ Manual ☐ Circuit

Type	Duration (min)	HR (min/max)	Dist / Floors	Intensity	Calories

Training Phase   Focus:

☐ Upper: _____
☐ Lower: _____
☐ Full/Combo: _____

Exercise	Set 1 (WU) reps / weight	Set 2 reps / weight	Set 3 reps / weight	Set 4 reps / weight	Set 5 reps / weight
1.	___x___	___x___	___x___	___x___	___x___
2.	___x___	___x___	___x___	___x___	___x___
3.	___x___	___x___	___x___	___x___	___x___
4.	___x___	___x___	___x___	___x___	___x___
5.	___x___	___x___	___x___	___x___	___x___
6.	___x___	___x___	___x___	___x___	___x___
7.	___x___	___x___	___x___	___x___	___x___
8.	___x___	___x___	___x___	___x___	___x___
9.	___x___	___x___	___x___	___x___	___x___
10.	___x___	___x___	___x___	___x___	___x___
11.	___x___	___x___	___x___	___x___	___x___
12.	___x___	___x___	___x___	___x___	___x___

Workout Comments:

Supplements:

Sleep (hrs): 1 2 3 4 5 6 7 8 9 10+   Workout Rating: 1 2 3 4 5 6 7 8 9 10

Partner/Trainer:_____   Date:_____
Injuries:_____   Time:_____ start / finish
BP/RHR/WT:_____   Location:_____

☐ Warm-up   ☐ Stretching   ☐ Cool-down

Cardio / Class Phase   Focus:

☐ Fat Burn   ☐ Random
☐ Interval   ☐ Bootcamp
☐ Manual   ☐ Circuit

Type	Duration (min)	HR (min/max)	Dist / Floors	Intensity	Calories

Training Phase   Focus:

☐ Upper: _____
☐ Lower: _____
☐ Full/Combo: _____

Exercise	Set 1 (WU) reps / weight	Set 2 reps / weight	Set 3 reps / weight	Set 4 reps / weight	Set 5 reps / weight
1.	___x___	___x___	___x___	___x___	___x___
2.	___x___	___x___	___x___	___x___	___x___
3.	___x___	___x___	___x___	___x___	___x___
4.	___x___	___x___	___x___	___x___	___x___
5.	___x___	___x___	___x___	___x___	___x___
6.	___x___	___x___	___x___	___x___	___x___
7.	___x___	___x___	___x___	___x___	___x___
8.	___x___	___x___	___x___	___x___	___x___
9.	___x___	___x___	___x___	___x___	___x___
10.	___x___	___x___	___x___	___x___	___x___
11.	___x___	___x___	___x___	___x___	___x___
12.	___x___	___x___	___x___	___x___	___x___

Workout Comments:

Supplements:

Sleep (hrs): 1 2 3 4 5 6 7 8 9 10+   Workout Rating: 1 2 3 4 5 6 7 8 9 10

Date:_____ Partner/Trainer:_____

Time:_____ start / finish _____ Injuries:_____

Location:_____ BP/RHR/WT:_____

☐ Warm-up ☐ Stretching ☐ Cool-down

Cardio / Class Phase **Focus:**

☐ Fat Burn ☐ Random
☐ Interval ☐ Bootcamp
☐ Manual ☐ Circuit

Type	Duration (min)	HR (min/max)	Dist / Floors	Intensity	Calories

Training Phase **Focus:**

☐ Upper: _____
☐ Lower: _____
☐ Full/Combo: _____

Exercise	Set 1 (WU) reps / weight	Set 2 reps / weight	Set 3 reps / weight	Set 4 reps / weight	Set 5 reps / weight
1.	__X__	__X__	__X__	__X__	__X__
2.	__X__	__X__	__X__	__X__	__X__
3.	__X__	__X__	__X__	__X__	__X__
4.	__X__	__X__	__X__	__X__	__X__
5.	__X__	__X__	__X__	__X__	__X__
6.	__X__	__X__	__X__	__X__	__X__
7.	__X__	__X__	__X__	__X__	__X__
8.	__X__	__X__	__X__	__X__	__X__
9.	__X__	__X__	__X__	__X__	__X__
10.	__X__	__X__	__X__	__X__	__X__
11.	__X__	__X__	__X__	__X__	__X__
12.	__X__	__X__	__X__	__X__	__X__

Workout Comments:

Supplements:

Sleep (hrs): 1 2 3 4 5 6 7 8 9 10+   Workout Rating: 1 2 3 4 5 6 7 8 9 10

Partner/Trainer:_____ Date:_____

Injuries:_____ Time:_____ start / finish _____

BP/RHR/WT:_____ Location:_____

☐ Warm-up ☐ Stretching ☐ Cool-down

Cardio / Class Phase   Focus:

☐ Fat Burn ☐ Random
☐ Interval ☐ Bootcamp
☐ Manual ☐ Circuit

Type	Duration (min)	HR (min/max)	Dist / Floors	Intensity	Calories

Training Phase   Focus:

☐ Upper: _____
☐ Lower: _____
☐ Full/Combo: _____

Exercise	Set 1 (WU) reps / weight	Set 2 reps / weight	Set 3 reps / weight	Set 4 reps / weight	Set 5 reps / weight
1.	____X____	____X____	____X____	____X____	____X____
2.	____X____	____X____	____X____	____X____	____X____
3.	____X____	____X____	____X____	____X____	____X____
4.	____X____	____X____	____X____	____X____	____X____
5.	____X____	____X____	____X____	____X____	____X____
6.	____X____	____X____	____X____	____X____	____X____
7.	____X____	____X____	____X____	____X____	____X____
8.	____X____	____X____	____X____	____X____	____X____
9.	____X____	____X____	____X____	____X____	____X____
10.	____X____	____X____	____X____	____X____	____X____
11.	____X____	____X____	____X____	____X____	____X____
12.	____X____	____X____	____X____	____X____	____X____

Workout Comments:

Supplements:

Sleep (hrs): 1 2 3 4 5 6 7 8 9 10+   Workout Rating: 1 2 3 4 5 6 7 8 9 10

Date:_____   Partner/Trainer:_____

Time:_____ start / finish _____   Injuries:_____

Location:_____   BP/RHR/WT:_____

☐ Warm-up ☐ Stretching ☐ Cool-down

Cardio / Class Phase   Focus:

☐ Fat Burn ☐ Random
☐ Interval ☐ Bootcamp
☐ Manual ☐ Circuit

Type	Duration (min)	HR (min/max)	Dist / Floors	Intensity	Calories

Training Phase   Focus:

☐ Upper: _____
☐ Lower: _____
☐ Full/Combo: _____

Exercise	Set 1 (WU) reps / weight	Set 2 reps / weight	Set 3 reps / weight	Set 4 reps / weight	Set 5 reps / weight
1.	___X___	___X___	___X___	___X___	___X___
2.	___X___	___X___	___X___	___X___	___X___
3.	___X___	___X___	___X___	___X___	___X___
4.	___X___	___X___	___X___	___X___	___X___
5.	___X___	___X___	___X___	___X___	___X___
6.	___X___	___X___	___X___	___X___	___X___
7.	___X___	___X___	___X___	___X___	___X___
8.	___X___	___X___	___X___	___X___	___X___
9.	___X___	___X___	___X___	___X___	___X___
10.	___X___	___X___	___X___	___X___	___X___
11.	___X___	___X___	___X___	___X___	___X___
12.	___X___	___X___	___X___	___X___	___X___

Workout Comments:

Supplements:

Sleep (hrs): 1 2 3 4 5 6 7 8 9 10+   Workout Rating: 1 2 3 4 5 6 7 8 9 10

Partner/Trainer:_____ Date:_____

Injuries:_____ Time:_____ start / finish _____

BP/RHR/WT:_____ Location:_____

☐ Warm-up ☐ Stretching ☐ Cool-down

Cardio / Class Phase

Focus:
☐ Fat Burn   ☐ Random
☐ Interval   ☐ Bootcamp
☐ Manual   ☐ Circuit

Type	Duration (min)	HR (min/max)	Dist / Floors	Intensity	Calories

Training Phase

Focus:
☐ Upper: _____
☐ Lower: _____
☐ Full/Combo: _____

Exercise	Set 1 (WU) reps / weight	Set 2 reps / weight	Set 3 reps / weight	Set 4 reps / weight	Set 5 reps / weight
1.	___X___	___X___	___X___	___X___	___X___
2.	___X___	___X___	___X___	___X___	___X___
3.	___X___	___X___	___X___	___X___	___X___
4.	___X___	___X___	___X___	___X___	___X___
5.	___X___	___X___	___X___	___X___	___X___
6.	___X___	___X___	___X___	___X___	___X___
7.	___X___	___X___	___X___	___X___	___X___
8.	___X___	___X___	___X___	___X___	___X___
9.	___X___	___X___	___X___	___X___	___X___
10.	___X___	___X___	___X___	___X___	___X___
11.	___X___	___X___	___X___	___X___	___X___
12.	___X___	___X___	___X___	___X___	___X___

Workout Comments:

Supplements:

Sleep (hrs): 1 2 3 4 5 6 7 8 9 10+   **Workout Rating:** 1 2 3 4 5 6 7 8 9 10

Date:_____   Partner/Trainer:_____

Time:_____ start / finish _____   Injuries:_____

Location:_____   BP/RHR/WT:_____

☐ Warm-up ☐ Stretching ☐ Cool-down

Cardio / Class Phase   Focus:

☐ Fat Burn ☐ Random
☐ Interval ☐ Bootcamp
☐ Manual   ☐ Circuit

Type	Duration (min)	HR (min/max)	Dist / Floors	Intensity	Calories

Training Phase   Focus:

☐ Upper: _____
☐ Lower: _____
☐ Full/Combo: _____

Exercise	Set 1 (WU) reps / weight	Set 2 reps / weight	Set 3 reps / weight	Set 4 reps / weight	Set 5 reps / weight
1.	___X___	___X___	___X___	___X___	___X___
2.	___X___	___X___	___X___	___X___	___X___
3.	___X___	___X___	___X___	___X___	___X___
4.	___X___	___X___	___X___	___X___	___X___
5.	___X___	___X___	___X___	___X___	___X___
6.	___X___	___X___	___X___	___X___	___X___
7.	___X___	___X___	___X___	___X___	___X___
8.	___X___	___X___	___X___	___X___	___X___
9.	___X___	___X___	___X___	___X___	___X___
10.	___X___	___X___	___X___	___X___	___X___
11.	___X___	___X___	___X___	___X___	___X___
12.	___X___	___X___	___X___	___X___	___X___

Workout Comments:

Supplements:

Sleep (hrs): 1 2 3 4 5 6 7 8 9 10+   Workout Rating: 1 2 3 4 5 6 7 8 9 10

Partner/Trainer:_____   Date:_____

Injuries:_____   Time:_____ start / finish _____

BP/RHR/WT:_____   Location:_____

☐ Warm-up   ☐ Stretching   ☐ Cool-down

Cardio / Class Phase   Focus:

☐ Fat Burn   ☐ Random
☐ Interval   ☐ Bootcamp
☐ Manual   ☐ Circuit

Type	Duration (min)	HR (min/max)	Dist / Floors	Intensity	Calories

Training Phase   Focus:

☐ Upper: _____
☐ Lower: _____
☐ Full/Combo: _____

Exercise	Set 1 (WU) reps / weight	Set 2 reps / weight	Set 3 reps / weight	Set 4 reps / weight	Set 5 reps / weight
1. ☐	___x___	___x___	___x___	___x___	___x___
2. ☐	___x___	___x___	___x___	___x___	___x___
3. ☐	___x___	___x___	___x___	___x___	___x___
4. ☐	___x___	___x___	___x___	___x___	___x___
5. ☐	___x___	___x___	___x___	___x___	___x___
6. ☐	___x___	___x___	___x___	___x___	___x___
7. ☐	___x___	___x___	___x___	___x___	___x___
8. ☐	___x___	___x___	___x___	___x___	___x___
9. ☐	___x___	___x___	___x___	___x___	___x___
10. ☐	___x___	___x___	___x___	___x___	___x___
11. ☐	___x___	___x___	___x___	___x___	___x___
12.	___x___	___x___	___x___	___x___	___x___

Workout Comments:

Supplements:

Sleep (hrs): 1 2 3 4 5 6 7 8 9 10+   Workout Rating: 1 2 3 4 5 6 7 8 9 10

Date:_____   Partner/Trainer:_____

Time:_____ start / finish   Injuries:_____

Location:_____   BP/RHR/WT:_____

□ Warm-up □ Stretching □ Cool-down

Cardio / Class Phase   Focus:

□ Fat Burn □ Random
□ Interval □ Bootcamp
□ Manual □ Circuit

Type	Duration (min)	HR (min/max)	Dist / Floors	Intensity	Calories

Training Phase   Focus:

□ Upper: _____
□ Lower: _____
□ Full/Combo: _____

Exercise	Set 1 (WU) reps / weight	Set 2 reps / weight	Set 3 reps / weight	Set 4 reps / weight	Set 5 reps / weight
1.	___ X ___	___ X ___	___ X ___	___ X ___	___ X ___
2.	___ X ___	___ X ___	___ X ___	___ X ___	___ X ___
3.	___ X ___	___ X ___	___ X ___	___ X ___	___ X ___
4.	___ X ___	___ X ___	___ X ___	___ X ___	___ X ___
5.	___ X ___	___ X ___	___ X ___	___ X ___	___ X ___
6.	___ X ___	___ X ___	___ X ___	___ X ___	___ X ___
7.	___ X ___	___ X ___	___ X ___	___ X ___	___ X ___
8.	___ X ___	___ X ___	___ X ___	___ X ___	___ X ___
9.	___ X ___	___ X ___	___ X ___	___ X ___	___ X ___
10.	___ X ___	___ X ___	___ X ___	___ X ___	___ X ___
11.	___ X ___	___ X ___	___ X ___	___ X ___	___ X ___
12.	___ X ___	___ X ___	___ X ___	___ X ___	___ X ___

Workout Comments:

Supplements:

Sleep (hrs): 1 2 3 4 5 6 7 8 9 10+   Workout Rating: 1 2 3 4 5 6 7 8 9 10

Partner/Trainer:_____

Injuries:_____

BP/RHR/WT:_____

Date:_____

Time:_____ start / finish _____

Location:_____

☐ Warm-up ☐ Stretching ☐ Cool-down

Cardio / Class Phase

Focus:
☐ Fat Burn ☐ Random
☐ Interval ☐ Bootcamp
☐ Manual ☐ Circuit

Type	Duration (min)	HR (min/max)	Dist / Floors	Intensity	Calories

Training Phase

Focus:
☐ Upper: _____
☐ Lower: _____
☐ Full/Combo: _____

Exercise	Set 1 (WU) reps / weight	Set 2 reps / weight	Set 3 reps / weight	Set 4 reps / weight	Set 5 reps / weight
1.	___X___	___X___	___X___	___X___	___X___
2.	___X___	___X___	___X___	___X___	___X___
3.	___X___	___X___	___X___	___X___	___X___
4.	___X___	___X___	___X___	___X___	___X___
5.	___X___	___X___	___X___	___X___	___X___
6.	___X___	___X___	___X___	___X___	___X___
7.	___X___	___X___	___X___	___X___	___X___
8.	___X___	___X___	___X___	___X___	___X___
9.	___X___	___X___	___X___	___X___	___X___
10.	___X___	___X___	___X___	___X___	___X___
11.	___X___	___X___	___X___	___X___	___X___
12.	___X___	___X___	___X___	___X___	___X___

Workout Comments:

Supplements:

Sleep (hrs): 1 2 3 4 5 6 7 8 9 10+   Workout Rating: 1 2 3 4 5 6 7 8 9 10

Date:_____   Partner/Trainer:_____

Time:_____   Injuries:_____
       start / finish

Location:_____   BP/RHR/WT:_____

☐ Warm-up   ☐ Stretching   ☐ Cool-down

Cardio / Class Phase   Focus:

☐ Fat Burn ☐ Random
☐ Interval ☐ Bootcamp
☐ Manual   ☐ Circuit

Type	Duration (min)	HR (min/max)	Dist / Floors	Intensity	Calories

Training Phase   Focus:

☐ Upper: _____
☐ Lower: _____
☐ Full/Combo: _____

Exercise	Set 1 (WU) reps / weight	Set 2 reps / weight	Set 3 reps / weight	Set 4 reps / weight	Set 5 reps / weight
1. ☐	___x___	___x___	___x___	___x___	___x___
2. ☐	___x___	___x___	___x___	___x___	___x___
3. ☐	___x___	___x___	___x___	___x___	___x___
4. ☐	___x___	___x___	___x___	___x___	___x___
5. ☐	___x___	___x___	___x___	___x___	___x___
6. ☐	___x___	___x___	___x___	___x___	___x___
7. ☐	___x___	___x___	___x___	___x___	___x___
8. ☐	___x___	___x___	___x___	___x___	___x___
9. ☐	___x___	___x___	___x___	___x___	___x___
10. ☐	___x___	___x___	___x___	___x___	___x___
11. ☐	___x___	___x___	___x___	___x___	___x___
12.	___x___	___x___	___x___	___x___	___x___

Workout Comments:

Supplements:

Sleep (hrs): 1 2 3 4 5 6 7 8 9 10+   Workout Rating: 1 2 3 4 5 6 7 8 9 10

Partner/Trainer:_____   Date:_____

Injuries:_____   Time:_____ start / finish

BP/RHR/WT:_____   Location:_____

☐ Warm-up   ☐ Stretching   ☐ Cool-down

Cardio / Class Phase   Focus:

☐ Fat Burn   ☐ Random
☐ Interval   ☐ Bootcamp
☐ Manual   ☐ Circuit

Type	Duration (min)	HR (min/max)	Dist / Floors	Intensity	Calories

Training Phase   Focus:

☐ Upper: _____
☐ Lower: _____
☐ Full/Combo: _____

Exercise	Set 1 (WU) reps / weight	Set 2 reps / weight	Set 3 reps / weight	Set 4 reps / weight	Set 5 reps / weight
1. ☐	___x___	___x___	___x___	___x___	___x___
2. ☐	___x___	___x___	___x___	___x___	___x___
3. ☐	___x___	___x___	___x___	___x___	___x___
4. ☐	___x___	___x___	___x___	___x___	___x___
5. ☐	___x___	___x___	___x___	___x___	___x___
6. ☐	___x___	___x___	___x___	___x___	___x___
7. ☐	___x___	___x___	___x___	___x___	___x___
8. ☐	___x___	___x___	___x___	___x___	___x___
9. ☐	___x___	___x___	___x___	___x___	___x___
10. ☐	___x___	___x___	___x___	___x___	___x___
11. ☐	___x___	___x___	___x___	___x___	___x___
12.	___x___	___x___	___x___	___x___	___x___

Workout Comments:

Supplements:

Sleep (hrs):   1   2   3   4   5   6   7   8   9   10+   Workout Rating: 1   2   3   4   5   6   7   8   9   10

Date:_____   Partner/Trainer:_____

Time:_____   Injuries:_____
start / finish

Location:_____   BP/RHR/WT:_____

☐ Warm-up ☐ Stretching ☐ Cool-down

Cardio / Class Phase

Focus:
☐ Fat Burn ☐ Random
☐ Interval ☐ Bootcamp
☐ Manual ☐ Circuit

Type	Duration (min)	HR (min/max)	Dist / Floors	Intensity	Calories

Training Phase

Focus:
☐ Upper: _____
☐ Lower: _____
☐ Full/Combo: _____

Exercise	Set 1 (WU) reps / weight	Set 2 reps / weight	Set 3 reps / weight	Set 4 reps / weight	Set 5 reps / weight
1.	___ X ___	___ X ___	___ X ___	___ X ___	___ X ___
2.	___ X ___	___ X ___	___ X ___	___ X ___	___ X ___
3.	___ X ___	___ X ___	___ X ___	___ X ___	___ X ___
4.	___ X ___	___ X ___	___ X ___	___ X ___	___ X ___
5.	___ X ___	___ X ___	___ X ___	___ X ___	___ X ___
6.	___ X ___	___ X ___	___ X ___	___ X ___	___ X ___
7.	___ X ___	___ X ___	___ X ___	___ X ___	___ X ___
8.	___ X ___	___ X ___	___ X ___	___ X ___	___ X ___
9.	___ X ___	___ X ___	___ X ___	___ X ___	___ X ___
10.	___ X ___	___ X ___	___ X ___	___ X ___	___ X ___
11.	___ X ___	___ X ___	___ X ___	___ X ___	___ X ___
12.	___ X ___	___ X ___	___ X ___	___ X ___	___ X ___

Workout Comments:

Supplements:

Sleep (hrs): 1 2 3 4 5 6 7 8 9 10+   Workout Rating: 1 2 3 4 5 6 7 8 9 10

Partner/Trainer:_____ Date:_____

Injuries:_____ Time:_____ start / finish _____

BP/RHR/WT:_____ Location:_____

☐ Warm-up ☐ Stretching ☐ Cool-down

Cardio / Class Phase

Focus:
☐ Fat Burn ☐ Random
☐ Interval ☐ Bootcamp
☐ Manual ☐ Circuit

Type	Duration (min)	HR (min/max)	Dist / Floors	Intensity	Calories

Training Phase

Focus:
☐ Upper: _____
☐ Lower: _____
☐ Full/Combo: _____

Exercise	Set 1 (WU) reps / weight	Set 2 reps / weight	Set 3 reps / weight	Set 4 reps / weight	Set 5 reps / weight
1.	___X___	___X___	___X___	___X___	___X___
2.	___X___	___X___	___X___	___X___	___X___
3.	___X___	___X___	___X___	___X___	___X___
4.	___X___	___X___	___X___	___X___	___X___
5.	___X___	___X___	___X___	___X___	___X___
6.	___X___	___X___	___X___	___X___	___X___
7.	___X___	___X___	___X___	___X___	___X___
8.	___X___	___X___	___X___	___X___	___X___
9.	___X___	___X___	___X___	___X___	___X___
10.	___X___	___X___	___X___	___X___	___X___
11.	___X___	___X___	___X___	___X___	___X___
12.	___X___	___X___	___X___	___X___	___X___

Workout Comments:

Supplements:

Sleep (hrs): 1 2 3 4 5 6 7 8 9 10+   Workout Rating: 1 2 3 4 5 6 7 8 9 10

Date:_____   Partner/Trainer:_____

Time:_____ start / finish _____   Injuries:_____

Location:_____   BP/RHR/WT:_____

☐ Warm-up ☐ Stretching ☐ Cool-down

Cardio / Class Phase   Focus:

☐ Fat Burn ☐ Random
☐ Interval ☐ Bootcamp
☐ Manual   ☐ Circuit

Type	Duration (min)	HR (min/max)	Dist / Floors	Intensity	Calories

Training Phase   Focus:

☐ Upper: _____
☐ Lower: _____
☐ Full/Combo: _____

Exercise	Set 1 (WU) reps / weight	Set 2 reps / weight	Set 3 reps / weight	Set 4 reps / weight	Set 5 reps / weight
1. ☐	___X___	___X___	___X___	___X___	___X___
2. ☐	___X___	___X___	___X___	___X___	___X___
3. ☐	___X___	___X___	___X___	___X___	___X___
4. ☐	___X___	___X___	___X___	___X___	___X___
5. ☐	___X___	___X___	___X___	___X___	___X___
6. ☐	___X___	___X___	___X___	___X___	___X___
7. ☐	___X___	___X___	___X___	___X___	___X___
8. ☐	___X___	___X___	___X___	___X___	___X___
9. ☐	___X___	___X___	___X___	___X___	___X___
10. ☐	___X___	___X___	___X___	___X___	___X___
11. ☐	___X___	___X___	___X___	___X___	___X___
12.	___X___	___X___	___X___	___X___	___X___

Workout Comments:

Supplements:

Sleep (hrs): 1 2 3 4 5 6 7 8 9 10+   Workout Rating: 1 2 3 4 5 6 7 8 9 10

Partner/Trainer:_____ Date:_____

Injuries:_____ Time:_____ start / finish

BP/RHR/WT:_____ Location:_____

☐ Warm-up   ☐ Stretching   ☐ Cool-down

Cardio / Class Phase   Focus:

☐ Fat Burn   ☐ Random
☐ Interval   ☐ Bootcamp
☐ Manual   ☐ Circuit

Type	Duration (min)	HR (min/max)	Dist / Floors	Intensity	Calories

Training Phase   Focus:

☐ Upper: _____
☐ Lower: _____
☐ Full/Combo: _____

Exercise	Set 1 (WU) reps / weight	Set 2 reps / weight	Set 3 reps / weight	Set 4 reps / weight	Set 5 reps / weight
1. ☐	____x____	____x____	____x____	____x____	____x____
2. ☐	____x____	____x____	____x____	____x____	____x____
3. ☐	____x____	____x____	____x____	____x____	____x____
4. ☐	____x____	____x____	____x____	____x____	____x____
5. ☐	____x____	____x____	____x____	____x____	____x____
6. ☐	____x____	____x____	____x____	____x____	____x____
7. ☐	____x____	____x____	____x____	____x____	____x____
8. ☐	____x____	____x____	____x____	____x____	____x____
9. ☐	____x____	____x____	____x____	____x____	____x____
10. ☐	____x____	____x____	____x____	____x____	____x____
11. ☐	____x____	____x____	____x____	____x____	____x____
12.	____x____	____x____	____x____	____x____	____x____

Workout Comments:

Supplements:

Sleep (hrs): 1 2 3 4 5 6 7 8 9 10+   Workout Rating: 1 2 3 4 5 6 7 8 9 10

Date:_____   Partner/Trainer:_____

Time:_____start / finish_____   Injuries:_____

Location:_____   BP/RHR/WT:_____

□ Warm-up   □ Stretching   □ Cool-down

Cardio / Class Phase   Focus:

□ Fat Burn   □ Random
□ Interval   □ Bootcamp
□ Manual   □ Circuit

Type	Duration (min)	HR (min/max)	Dist / Floors	Intensity	Calories

Training Phase   Focus:

□ Upper: _____
□ Lower: _____
□ Full/Combo: _____

Exercise	Set 1 (WU) reps / weight	Set 2 reps / weight	Set 3 reps / weight	Set 4 reps / weight	Set 5 reps / weight
1. □	___X___	___X___	___X___	___X___	___X___
2. □	___X___	___X___	___X___	___X___	___X___
3. □	___X___	___X___	___X___	___X___	___X___
4. □	___X___	___X___	___X___	___X___	___X___
5. □	___X___	___X___	___X___	___X___	___X___
6. □	___X___	___X___	___X___	___X___	___X___
7. □	___X___	___X___	___X___	___X___	___X___
8. □	___X___	___X___	___X___	___X___	___X___
9. □	___X___	___X___	___X___	___X___	___X___
10. □	___X___	___X___	___X___	___X___	___X___
11. □	___X___	___X___	___X___	___X___	___X___
12.	___X___	___X___	___X___	___X___	___X___

Workout Comments:

Supplements:

Sleep (hrs): 1 2 3 4 5 6 7 8 9 10+   Workout Rating: 1 2 3 4 5 6 7 8 9 10

Partner/Trainer:_____ Date:_____

Injuries:_____ Time:_____ start / finish _____

BP/RHR/WT:_____ Location:_____

☐ Warm-up ☐ Stretching ☐ Cool-down

Cardio / Class Phase

Focus:
☐ Fat Burn ☐ Random
☐ Interval ☐ Bootcamp
☐ Manual ☐ Circuit

Type	Duration (min)	HR (min/max)	Dist / Floors	Intensity	Calories

Training Phase

Focus:
☐ Upper: _____
☐ Lower: _____
☐ Full/Combo: _____

Exercise	Set 1 (WU) reps / weight	Set 2 reps / weight	Set 3 reps / weight	Set 4 reps / weight	Set 5 reps / weight
1.	___X___	___X___	___X___	___X___	___X___
2.	___X___	___X___	___X___	___X___	___X___
3.	___X___	___X___	___X___	___X___	___X___
4.	___X___	___X___	___X___	___X___	___X___
5.	___X___	___X___	___X___	___X___	___X___
6.	___X___	___X___	___X___	___X___	___X___
7.	___X___	___X___	___X___	___X___	___X___
8.	___X___	___X___	___X___	___X___	___X___
9.	___X___	___X___	___X___	___X___	___X___
10.	___X___	___X___	___X___	___X___	___X___
11.	___X___	___X___	___X___	___X___	___X___
12.	___X___	___X___	___X___	___X___	___X___

Workout Comments:

Supplements:

Sleep (hrs): 1 2 3 4 5 6 7 8 9 10+   Workout Rating: 1 2 3 4 5 6 7 8 9 10

Date:_____ Partner/Trainer:_____

Time:_____ start / finish _____ Injuries:_____

Location:_____ BP/RHR/WT:_____

□ Warm-up   □ Stretching   □ Cool-down

Cardio / Class Phase   Focus:

□ Fat Burn   □ Random
□ Interval   □ Bootcamp
□ Manual   □ Circuit

Type	Duration (min)	HR (min/max)	Dist / Floors	Intensity	Calories

Training Phase   Focus:

□ Upper: _____
□ Lower: _____
□ Full/Combo: _____

Exercise	Set 1 (WU) reps / weight	Set 2 reps / weight	Set 3 reps / weight	Set 4 reps / weight	Set 5 reps / weight
1.	___X___	___X___	___X___	___X___	___X___
2.	___X___	___X___	___X___	___X___	___X___
3.	___X___	___X___	___X___	___X___	___X___
4.	___X___	___X___	___X___	___X___	___X___
5.	___X___	___X___	___X___	___X___	___X___
6.	___X___	___X___	___X___	___X___	___X___
7.	___X___	___X___	___X___	___X___	___X___
8.	___X___	___X___	___X___	___X___	___X___
9.	___X___	___X___	___X___	___X___	___X___
10.	___X___	___X___	___X___	___X___	___X___
11.	___X___	___X___	___X___	___X___	___X___
12.	___X___	___X___	___X___	___X___	___X___

Workout Comments:

Supplements:

Sleep (hrs): 1 2 3 4 5 6 7 8 9 10+   Workout Rating: 1 2 3 4 5 6 7 8 9 10

Partner/Trainer:_____ Date:_____

Injuries:_____ Time:_____ start / finish

BP/RHR/WT:_____ Location:_____

☐ Warm-up ☐ Stretching ☐ Cool-down

Cardio / Class Phase

Focus:

☐ Fat Burn ☐ Random
☐ Interval ☐ Bootcamp
☐ Manual   ☐ Circuit

Type	Duration (min)	HR (min/max)	Dist / Floors	Intensity	Calories

Training Phase

Focus:
☐ Upper: _____
☐ Lower: _____
☐ Full/Combo: _____

Exercise	Set 1 (WU) reps / weight	Set 2 reps / weight	Set 3 reps / weight	Set 4 reps / weight	Set 5 reps / weight
1.	___x___	___x___	___x___	___x___	___x___
2.	___x___	___x___	___x___	___x___	___x___
3.	___x___	___x___	___x___	___x___	___x___
4.	___x___	___x___	___x___	___x___	___x___
5.	___x___	___x___	___x___	___x___	___x___
6.	___x___	___x___	___x___	___x___	___x___
7.	___x___	___x___	___x___	___x___	___x___
8.	___x___	___x___	___x___	___x___	___x___
9.	___x___	___x___	___x___	___x___	___x___
10.	___x___	___x___	___x___	___x___	___x___
11.	___x___	___x___	___x___	___x___	___x___
12.	___x___	___x___	___x___	___x___	___x___

Workout Comments:

Supplements:

Sleep (hrs): 1 2 3 4 5 6 7 8 9 10+   Workout Rating: 1 2 3 4 5 6 7 8 9 10

Date:_____ Partner/Trainer:_____

Time:_____ start / finish _____ Injuries:_____

Location:_____ BP/RHR/WT:_____

☐ Warm-up ☐ Stretching ☐ Cool-down

Cardio / Class Phase Focus:

☐ Fat Burn ☐ Random
☐ Interval ☐ Bootcamp
☐ Manual ☐ Circuit

Type	Duration (min)	HR (min/max)	Dist / Floors	Intensity	Calories

Training Phase Focus:

☐ Upper: _____
☐ Lower: _____
☐ Full/Combo: _____

Exercise	Set 1 (WU) reps / weight	Set 2 reps / weight	Set 3 reps / weight	Set 4 reps / weight	Set 5 reps / weight
1.	___X___	___X___	___X___	___X___	___X___
2.	___X___	___X___	___X___	___X___	___X___
3.	___X___	___X___	___X___	___X___	___X___
4.	___X___	___X___	___X___	___X___	___X___
5.	___X___	___X___	___X___	___X___	___X___
6.	___X___	___X___	___X___	___X___	___X___
7.	___X___	___X___	___X___	___X___	___X___
8.	___X___	___X___	___X___	___X___	___X___
9.	___X___	___X___	___X___	___X___	___X___
10.	___X___	___X___	___X___	___X___	___X___
11.	___X___	___X___	___X___	___X___	___X___
12.	___X___	___X___	___X___	___X___	___X___

Workout Comments:

Supplements:

Sleep (hrs): 1 2 3 4 5 6 7 8 9 10+   Workout Rating: 1 2 3 4 5 6 7 8 9 10

Partner/Trainer:_____

Injuries:_____

BP/RHR/WT:_____

Date:_____

Time:_____ start / finish

Location:_____

☐ Warm-up ☐ Stretching ☐ Cool-down

Cardio / Class Phase

Focus:
☐ Fat Burn ☐ Random
☐ Interval ☐ Bootcamp
☐ Manual ☐ Circuit

Type	Duration (min)	HR (min/max)	Dist / Floors	Intensity	Calories

Training Phase

Focus:
☐ Upper: _____
☐ Lower: _____
☐ Full/Combo: _____

Exercise	Set 1 (WU) reps / weight	Set 2 reps / weight	Set 3 reps / weight	Set 4 reps / weight	Set 5 reps / weight
1. ☐	___X___	___X___	___X___	___X___	___X___
2. ☐	___X___	___X___	___X___	___X___	___X___
3. ☐	___X___	___X___	___X___	___X___	___X___
4. ☐	___X___	___X___	___X___	___X___	___X___
5. ☐	___X___	___X___	___X___	___X___	___X___
6. ☐	___X___	___X___	___X___	___X___	___X___
7. ☐	___X___	___X___	___X___	___X___	___X___
8. ☐	___X___	___X___	___X___	___X___	___X___
9. ☐	___X___	___X___	___X___	___X___	___X___
10. ☐	___X___	___X___	___X___	___X___	___X___
11. ☐	___X___	___X___	___X___	___X___	___X___
12.	___X___	___X___	___X___	___X___	___X___

Workout Comments:

Supplements:

Sleep (hrs): 1 2 3 4 5 6 7 8 9 10+   Workout Rating: 1 2 3 4 5 6 7 8 9 10

Date:_____   Partner/Trainer:_____

Time:_____ start / finish _____   Injuries:_____

Location:_____   BP/RHR/WT:_____

☐ Warm-up ☐ Stretching ☐ Cool-down

Cardio / Class Phase

Focus:
☐ Fat Burn ☐ Random
☐ Interval ☐ Bootcamp
☐ Manual ☐ Circuit

Type	Duration (min)	HR (min/max)	Dist / Floors	Intensity	Calories

Training Phase

Focus:
☐ Upper: _____
☐ Lower: _____
☐ Full/Combo: _____

Exercise	Set 1 (WU) reps / weight	Set 2 reps / weight	Set 3 reps / weight	Set 4 reps / weight	Set 5 reps / weight
1. ☐	___X___	___X___	___X___	___X___	___X___
2. ☐	___X___	___X___	___X___	___X___	___X___
3. ☐	___X___	___X___	___X___	___X___	___X___
4. ☐	___X___	___X___	___X___	___X___	___X___
5. ☐	___X___	___X___	___X___	___X___	___X___
6. ☐	___X___	___X___	___X___	___X___	___X___
7. ☐	___X___	___X___	___X___	___X___	___X___
8. ☐	___X___	___X___	___X___	___X___	___X___
9. ☐	___X___	___X___	___X___	___X___	___X___
10. ☐	___X___	___X___	___X___	___X___	___X___
11. ☐	___X___	___X___	___X___	___X___	___X___
12.	___X___	___X___	___X___	___X___	___X___

Workout Comments:

Supplements:

Sleep (hrs): 1 2 3 4 5 6 7 8 9 10+   Workout Rating: 1 2 3 4 5 6 7 8 9 10

Partner/Trainer:_____   Date:_____

Injuries:_____   Time:_____ start / finish _____

BP/RHR/WT:_____   Location:_____

□ Warm-up   □ Stretching   □ Cool-down

Cardio / Class Phase   Focus:

□ Fat Burn   □ Random
□ Interval   □ Bootcamp
□ Manual   □ Circuit

Type	Duration (min)	HR (min/max)	Dist / Floors	Intensity	Calories

Training Phase   Focus:

□ Upper: _____
□ Lower: _____
□ Full/Combo: _____

Exercise	Set 1 (WU) reps / weight	Set 2 reps / weight	Set 3 reps / weight	Set 4 reps / weight	Set 5 reps / weight
1.	___X___	___X___	___X___	___X___	___X___
2.	___X___	___X___	___X___	___X___	___X___
3.	___X___	___X___	___X___	___X___	___X___
4.	___X___	___X___	___X___	___X___	___X___
5.	___X___	___X___	___X___	___X___	___X___
6.	___X___	___X___	___X___	___X___	___X___
7.	___X___	___X___	___X___	___X___	___X___
8.	___X___	___X___	___X___	___X___	___X___
9.	___X___	___X___	___X___	___X___	___X___
10.	___X___	___X___	___X___	___X___	___X___
11.	___X___	___X___	___X___	___X___	___X___
12.	___X___	___X___	___X___	___X___	___X___

Workout Comments:

Supplements:

Sleep (hrs): 1 2 3 4 5 6 7 8 9 10+   Workout Rating: 1 2 3 4 5 6 7 8 9 10

Date:_____   Partner/Trainer:_____

Time:_____ start / finish   Injuries:_____

Location:_____   BP/RHR/WT:_____

☐ Warm-up   ☐ Stretching   ☐ Cool-down

Cardio / Class Phase   Focus:

☐ Fat Burn   ☐ Random
☐ Interval   ☐ Bootcamp
☐ Manual   ☐ Circuit

Type	Duration (min)	HR (min/max)	Dist / Floors	Intensity	Calories

Training Phase   Focus:

☐ Upper: _____
☐ Lower: _____
☐ Full/Combo: _____

Exercise	Set 1 (WU) reps / weight	Set 2 reps / weight	Set 3 reps / weight	Set 4 reps / weight	Set 5 reps / weight
1.	___x___	___x___	___x___	___x___	___x___
2.	___x___	___x___	___x___	___x___	___x___
3.	___x___	___x___	___x___	___x___	___x___
4.	___x___	___x___	___x___	___x___	___x___
5.	___x___	___x___	___x___	___x___	___x___
6.	___x___	___x___	___x___	___x___	___x___
7.	___x___	___x___	___x___	___x___	___x___
8.	___x___	___x___	___x___	___x___	___x___
9.	___x___	___x___	___x___	___x___	___x___
10.	___x___	___x___	___x___	___x___	___x___
11.	___x___	___x___	___x___	___x___	___x___
12.	___x___	___x___	___x___	___x___	___x___

Workout Comments:

Supplements:

Sleep (hrs): 1 2 3 4 5 6 7 8 9 10+   Workout Rating: 1 2 3 4 5 6 7 8 9 10

Partner/Trainer:_____ Date:_____

Injuries:_____ Time:_____ start / finish _____

BP/RHR/WT:_____ Location:_____

☐ Warm-up ☐ Stretching ☐ Cool-down

Cardio / Class Phase   Focus:

☐ Fat Burn ☐ Random
☐ Interval ☐ Bootcamp
☐ Manual   ☐ Circuit

Type	Duration (min)	HR (min/max)	Dist / Floors	Intensity	Calories

Training Phase   Focus:

☐ Upper: _____
☐ Lower: _____
☐ Full/Combo: _____

Exercise	Set 1 (WU) reps / weight	Set 2 reps / weight	Set 3 reps / weight	Set 4 reps / weight	Set 5 reps / weight
1.	___X___	___X___	___X___	___X___	___X___
2.	___X___	___X___	___X___	___X___	___X___
3.	___X___	___X___	___X___	___X___	___X___
4.	___X___	___X___	___X___	___X___	___X___
5.	___X___	___X___	___X___	___X___	___X___
6.	___X___	___X___	___X___	___X___	___X___
7.	___X___	___X___	___X___	___X___	___X___
8.	___X___	___X___	___X___	___X___	___X___
9.	___X___	___X___	___X___	___X___	___X___
10.	___X___	___X___	___X___	___X___	___X___
11.	___X___	___X___	___X___	___X___	___X___
12.	___X___	___X___	___X___	___X___	___X___

Workout Comments:

Supplements:

Sleep (hrs): 1 2 3 4 5 6 7 8 9 10+   Workout Rating: 1 2 3 4 5 6 7 8 9 10

Date:_____   Partner/Trainer:_____

Time:_____   Injuries:_____
        start / finish

Location:_____   BP/RHR/WT:_____

☐ Warm-up ☐ Stretching ☐ Cool-down

Cardio / Class Phase

Focus:
☐ Fat Burn ☐ Random
☐ Interval ☐ Bootcamp
☐ Manual ☐ Circuit

Type	Duration (min)	HR (min/max)	Dist / Floors	Intensity	Calories

Training Phase

Focus:
☐ Upper: _____
☐ Lower: _____
☐ Full/Combo: _____

Exercise	Set 1 (WU) reps / weight	Set 2 reps / weight	Set 3 reps / weight	Set 4 reps / weight	Set 5 reps / weight
1.	___ X ___	___ X ___	___ X ___	___ X ___	___ X ___
2.	___ X ___	___ X ___	___ X ___	___ X ___	___ X ___
3.	___ X ___	___ X ___	___ X ___	___ X ___	___ X ___
4.	___ X ___	___ X ___	___ X ___	___ X ___	___ X ___
5.	___ X ___	___ X ___	___ X ___	___ X ___	___ X ___
6.	___ X ___	___ X ___	___ X ___	___ X ___	___ X ___
7.	___ X ___	___ X ___	___ X ___	___ X ___	___ X ___
8.	___ X ___	___ X ___	___ X ___	___ X ___	___ X ___
9.	___ X ___	___ X ___	___ X ___	___ X ___	___ X ___
10.	___ X ___	___ X ___	___ X ___	___ X ___	___ X ___
11.	___ X ___	___ X ___	___ X ___	___ X ___	___ X ___
12.	___ X ___	___ X ___	___ X ___	___ X ___	___ X ___

Workout Comments:

Supplements:

Sleep (hrs): 1 2 3 4 5 6 7 8 9 10+   Workout Rating: 1 2 3 4 5 6 7 8 9 10

Partner/Trainer:_____ Date:_____

Injuries:_____ Time:_____ start / finish _____

BP/RHR/WT:_____ Location:_____

☐ Warm-up ☐ Stretching ☐ Cool-down

Cardio / Class Phase

Focus:
☐ Fat Burn ☐ Random
☐ Interval ☐ Bootcamp
☐ Manual ☐ Circuit

Type	Duration (min)	HR (min/max)	Dist / Floors	Intensity	Calories

Training Phase

Focus:
☐ Upper: _____
☐ Lower: _____
☐ Full/Combo: _____

Exercise	Set 1 (WU) reps / weight	Set 2 reps / weight	Set 3 reps / weight	Set 4 reps / weight	Set 5 reps / weight
1.	___x___	___x___	___x___	___x___	___x___
2.	___x___	___x___	___x___	___x___	___x___
3.	___x___	___x___	___x___	___x___	___x___
4.	___x___	___x___	___x___	___x___	___x___
5.	___x___	___x___	___x___	___x___	___x___
6.	___x___	___x___	___x___	___x___	___x___
7.	___x___	___x___	___x___	___x___	___x___
8.	___x___	___x___	___x___	___x___	___x___
9.	___x___	___x___	___x___	___x___	___x___
10.	___x___	___x___	___x___	___x___	___x___
11.	___x___	___x___	___x___	___x___	___x___
12.	___x___	___x___	___x___	___x___	___x___

Workout Comments:

Supplements:

Sleep (hrs): 1 2 3 4 5 6 7 8 9 10+   Workout Rating: 1 2 3 4 5 6 7 8 9 10

Date:_____   Partner/Trainer:_____

Time:_____   Injuries:_____
start / finish

Location:_____   BP/RHR/WT:_____

☐ Warm-up ☐ Stretching ☐ Cool-down

Cardio / Class Phase   Focus:

☐ Fat Burn ☐ Random
☐ Interval ☐ Bootcamp
☐ Manual ☐ Circuit

Type	Duration (min)	HR (min/max)	Dist / Floors	Intensity	Calories

Training Phase   Focus:

☐ Upper: _____
☐ Lower: _____
☐ Full/Combo: _____

Exercise	Set 1 (WU) reps / weight	Set 2 reps / weight	Set 3 reps / weight	Set 4 reps / weight	Set 5 reps / weight
1. ☐	___X___	___X___	___X___	___X___	___X___
2. ☐	___X___	___X___	___X___	___X___	___X___
3. ☐	___X___	___X___	___X___	___X___	___X___
4. ☐	___X___	___X___	___X___	___X___	___X___
5. ☐	___X___	___X___	___X___	___X___	___X___
6. ☐	___X___	___X___	___X___	___X___	___X___
7. ☐	___X___	___X___	___X___	___X___	___X___
8. ☐	___X___	___X___	___X___	___X___	___X___
9. ☐	___X___	___X___	___X___	___X___	___X___
10. ☐	___X___	___X___	___X___	___X___	___X___
11. ☐	___X___	___X___	___X___	___X___	___X___
12. ☐	___X___	___X___	___X___	___X___	___X___

Workout Comments:

Supplements:

Sleep (hrs): 1 2 3 4 5 6 7 8 9 10+   Workout Rating: 1 2 3 4 5 6 7 8 9 10

Partner/Trainer:_____

Injuries:_____

BP/RHR/WT:_____

Date:_____

Time:_____ start / finish _____

Location:_____

□ Warm-up □ Stretching □ Cool-down

Cardio / Class Phase

Focus:
□ Fat Burn □ Random
□ Interval □ Bootcamp
□ Manual □ Circuit

Type	Duration (min)	HR (min/max)	Dist / Floors	Intensity	Calories

Training Phase

Focus:
□ Upper: _____
□ Lower: _____
□ Full/Combo: _____

Exercise	Set 1 (WU) reps / weight	Set 2 reps / weight	Set 3 reps / weight	Set 4 reps / weight	Set 5 reps / weight
1.	___x___	___x___	___x___	___x___	___x___
2.	___x___	___x___	___x___	___x___	___x___
3.	___x___	___x___	___x___	___x___	___x___
4.	___x___	___x___	___x___	___x___	___x___
5.	___x___	___x___	___x___	___x___	___x___
6.	___x___	___x___	___x___	___x___	___x___
7.	___x___	___x___	___x___	___x___	___x___
8.	___x___	___x___	___x___	___x___	___x___
9.	___x___	___x___	___x___	___x___	___x___
10.	___x___	___x___	___x___	___x___	___x___
11.	___x___	___x___	___x___	___x___	___x___
12.	___x___	___x___	___x___	___x___	___x___

Workout Comments:

Supplements:

Sleep (hrs): 1 2 3 4 5 6 7 8 9 10+   Workout Rating: 1 2 3 4 5 6 7 8 9 10

Date:	Partner/Trainer:
Time: _____ start / finish _____	Injuries:
Location:	BP/RHR/WT:

☐ Warm-up ☐ Stretching ☐ Cool-down

Cardio / Class Phase   Focus:

☐ Fat Burn ☐ Random
☐ Interval ☐ Bootcamp
☐ Manual   ☐ Circuit

Type	Duration (min)	HR (min/max)	Dist / Floors	Intensity	Calories

Training Phase   Focus:

☐ Upper: _____
☐ Lower: _____
☐ Full/Combo: _____

Exercise	Set 1 (WU) reps / weight	Set 2 reps / weight	Set 3 reps / weight	Set 4 reps / weight	Set 5 reps / weight
1.	___x___	___x___	___x___	___x___	___x___
2.	___x___	___x___	___x___	___x___	___x___
3.	___x___	___x___	___x___	___x___	___x___
4.	___x___	___x___	___x___	___x___	___x___
5.	___x___	___x___	___x___	___x___	___x___
6.	___x___	___x___	___x___	___x___	___x___
7.	___x___	___x___	___x___	___x___	___x___
8.	___x___	___x___	___x___	___x___	___x___
9.	___x___	___x___	___x___	___x___	___x___
10.	___x___	___x___	___x___	___x___	___x___
11.	___x___	___x___	___x___	___x___	___x___
12.	___x___	___x___	___x___	___x___	___x___

Workout Comments:

Supplements:

Sleep (hrs): 1 2 3 4 5 6 7 8 9 10+   Workout Rating: 1 2 3 4 5 6 7 8 9 10

Partner/Trainer:_____ Date:_____

Injuries:_____ Time:_____ start / finish _____

BP/RHR/WT:_____ Location:_____

☐ Warm-up   ☐ Stretching   ☐ Cool-down

Cardio / Class Phase

Focus:
☐ Fat Burn   ☐ Random
☐ Interval   ☐ Bootcamp
☐ Manual   ☐ Circuit

Type	Duration (min)	HR (min/max)	Dist / Floors	Intensity	Calories

Training Phase

Focus:
☐ Upper: _____
☐ Lower: _____
☐ Full/Combo: _____

Exercise	Set 1 (WU) reps / weight	Set 2 reps / weight	Set 3 reps / weight	Set 4 reps / weight	Set 5 reps / weight
1. ☐	___ X ___	___ X ___	___ X ___	___ X ___	___ X ___
2. ☐	___ X ___	___ X ___	___ X ___	___ X ___	___ X ___
3. ☐	___ X ___	___ X ___	___ X ___	___ X ___	___ X ___
4. ☐	___ X ___	___ X ___	___ X ___	___ X ___	___ X ___
5. ☐	___ X ___	___ X ___	___ X ___	___ X ___	___ X ___
6. ☐	___ X ___	___ X ___	___ X ___	___ X ___	___ X ___
7. ☐	___ X ___	___ X ___	___ X ___	___ X ___	___ X ___
8. ☐	___ X ___	___ X ___	___ X ___	___ X ___	___ X ___
9. ☐	___ X ___	___ X ___	___ X ___	___ X ___	___ X ___
10. ☐	___ X ___	___ X ___	___ X ___	___ X ___	___ X ___
11. ☐	___ X ___	___ X ___	___ X ___	___ X ___	___ X ___
12.	___ X ___	___ X ___	___ X ___	___ X ___	___ X ___

Workout Comments:

Supplements:

Sleep (hrs): 1 2 3 4 5 6 7 8 9 10+   Workout Rating: 1 2 3 4 5 6 7 8 9 10

Date:_____   Partner/Trainer:_____

Time:_____   Injuries:_____
       start / finish

Location:_____   BP/RHR/WT:_____

☐ Warm-up   ☐ Stretching   ☐ Cool-down

Cardio / Class Phase   Focus:

	☐ Fat Burn	☐ Random
☐ Interval	☐ Bootcamp
☐ Manual	☐ Circuit

Type	Duration (min)	HR (min/max)	Dist / Floors	Intensity	Calories

Training Phase   Focus:

☐ Upper: _____
☐ Lower: _____
☐ Full/Combo: _____

Exercise	Set 1 (WU) reps / weight	Set 2 reps / weight	Set 3 reps / weight	Set 4 reps / weight	Set 5 reps / weight
1. ☐	___X___	___X___	___X___	___X___	___X___
2. ☐	___X___	___X___	___X___	___X___	___X___
3. ☐	___X___	___X___	___X___	___X___	___X___
4. ☐	___X___	___X___	___X___	___X___	___X___
5. ☐	___X___	___X___	___X___	___X___	___X___
6. ☐	___X___	___X___	___X___	___X___	___X___
7. ☐	___X___	___X___	___X___	___X___	___X___
8. ☐	___X___	___X___	___X___	___X___	___X___
9. ☐	___X___	___X___	___X___	___X___	___X___
10. ☐	___X___	___X___	___X___	___X___	___X___
11. ☐	___X___	___X___	___X___	___X___	___X___
12.	___X___	___X___	___X___	___X___	___X___

Workout Comments:

Supplements:

Sleep (hrs): 1 2 3 4 5 6 7 8 9 10+   Workout Rating: 1 2 3 4 5 6 7 8 9 10

Partner/Trainer:_____   Date:_____

Injuries:_____   Time:_____ start / finish ____

BP/RHR/WT:_____   Location:_____

☐ Warm-up ☐ Stretching ☐ Cool-down

Cardio / Class Phase   Focus:

☐ Fat Burn   ☐ Random
☐ Interval   ☐ Bootcamp
☐ Manual   ☐ Circuit

Type	Duration (min)	HR (min/max)	Dist / Floors	Intensity	Calories

Training Phase   Focus:

☐ Upper: _____
☐ Lower: _____
☐ Full/Combo: _____

Exercise	Set 1 (WU) reps / weight	Set 2 reps / weight	Set 3 reps / weight	Set 4 reps / weight	Set 5 reps / weight
1.	___x___	___x___	___x___	___x___	___x___
2.	___x___	___x___	___x___	___x___	___x___
3.	___x___	___x___	___x___	___x___	___x___
4.	___x___	___x___	___x___	___x___	___x___
5.	___x___	___x___	___x___	___x___	___x___
6.	___x___	___x___	___x___	___x___	___x___
7.	___x___	___x___	___x___	___x___	___x___
8.	___x___	___x___	___x___	___x___	___x___
9.	___x___	___x___	___x___	___x___	___x___
10.	___x___	___x___	___x___	___x___	___x___
11.	___x___	___x___	___x___	___x___	___x___
12.	___x___	___x___	___x___	___x___	___x___

Workout Comments:

Supplements:

Sleep (hrs): 1 2 3 4 5 6 7 8 9 10+   Workout Rating: 1 2 3 4 5 6 7 8 9 10

Date:_____ Partner/Trainer:_____

Time:_____ start / finish Injuries:_____

Location:_____ BP/RHR/WT:_____

☐ Warm-up ☐ Stretching ☐ Cool-down

Cardio / Class Phase

Focus:
☐ Fat Burn ☐ Random
☐ Interval ☐ Bootcamp
☐ Manual ☐ Circuit

Type	Duration (min)	HR (min/max)	Dist / Floors	Intensity	Calories

Training Phase

Focus:
☐ Upper: _____
☐ Lower: _____
☐ Full/Combo: _____

Exercise	Set 1 (WU) reps / weight	Set 2 reps / weight	Set 3 reps / weight	Set 4 reps / weight	Set 5 reps / weight
1.	___X___	___X___	___X___	___X___	___X___
2.	___X___	___X___	___X___	___X___	___X___
3.	___X___	___X___	___X___	___X___	___X___
4.	___X___	___X___	___X___	___X___	___X___
5.	___X___	___X___	___X___	___X___	___X___
6.	___X___	___X___	___X___	___X___	___X___
7.	___X___	___X___	___X___	___X___	___X___
8.	___X___	___X___	___X___	___X___	___X___
9.	___X___	___X___	___X___	___X___	___X___
10.	___X___	___X___	___X___	___X___	___X___
11.	___X___	___X___	___X___	___X___	___X___
12.	___X___	___X___	___X___	___X___	___X___

Workout Comments:

Supplements:

Sleep (hrs): 1 2 3 4 5 6 7 8 9 10+   Workout Rating: 1 2 3 4 5 6 7 8 9 10

Partner/Trainer: _____	Date: _____
Injuries: _____	Time: _____ start / finish _____
BP/RHR/WT: _____	Location: _____

☐ Warm-up　☐ Stretching　☐ Cool-down

Cardio / Class Phase　Focus:

☐ Fat Burn　☐ Random
☐ Interval　☐ Bootcamp
☐ Manual　☐ Circuit

Type	Duration (min)	HR (min/max)	Dist / Floors	Intensity	Calories

Training Phase　Focus:

☐ Upper: _____
☐ Lower: _____
☐ Full/Combo: _____

Exercise	Set 1 (WU) reps / weight	Set 2 reps / weight	Set 3 reps / weight	Set 4 reps / weight	Set 5 reps / weight
1.	____X____	____X____	____X____	____X____	____X____
2.	____X____	____X____	____X____	____X____	____X____
3.	____X____	____X____	____X____	____X____	____X____
4.	____X____	____X____	____X____	____X____	____X____
5.	____X____	____X____	____X____	____X____	____X____
6.	____X____	____X____	____X____	____X____	____X____
7.	____X____	____X____	____X____	____X____	____X____
8.	____X____	____X____	____X____	____X____	____X____
9.	____X____	____X____	____X____	____X____	____X____
10.	____X____	____X____	____X____	____X____	____X____
11.	____X____	____X____	____X____	____X____	____X____
12.	____X____	____X____	____X____	____X____	____X____

Workout Comments:

Supplements:

Sleep (hrs):　1　2　3　4　5　6　7　8　9　10+　　Workout Rating:　1　2　3　4　5　6　7　8　9　10

Date:_____ Partner/Trainer:_____

Time:_____start / finish_____ Injuries:_____

Location:_____ BP/RHR/WT:_____

☐ Warm-up ☐ Stretching ☐ Cool-down

Cardio / Class Phase   Focus:

☐ Fat Burn ☐ Random
☐ Interval ☐ Bootcamp
☐ Manual ☐ Circuit

Type	Duration (min)	HR (min/max)	Dist / Floors	Intensity	Calories

Training Phase   Focus:

☐ Upper: _____
☐ Lower: _____
☐ Full/Combo: _____

Exercise	Set 1 (WU) reps / weight	Set 2 reps / weight	Set 3 reps / weight	Set 4 reps / weight	Set 5 reps / weight
1. ☐	___X___	___X___	___X___	___X___	___X___
2. ☐	___X___	___X___	___X___	___X___	___X___
3. ☐	___X___	___X___	___X___	___X___	___X___
4. ☐	___X___	___X___	___X___	___X___	___X___
5. ☐	___X___	___X___	___X___	___X___	___X___
6. ☐	___X___	___X___	___X___	___X___	___X___
7. ☐	___X___	___X___	___X___	___X___	___X___
8. ☐	___X___	___X___	___X___	___X___	___X___
9. ☐	___X___	___X___	___X___	___X___	___X___
10. ☐	___X___	___X___	___X___	___X___	___X___
11. ☐	___X___	___X___	___X___	___X___	___X___
12.	___X___	___X___	___X___	___X___	___X___

Workout Comments:

Supplements:

Sleep (hrs): 1 2 3 4 5 6 7 8 9 10+   Workout Rating: 1 2 3 4 5 6 7 8 9 10

My Nutrition Log

21 Day Challenge #1

21-Day Kick Start Eating Challenge
7 Simple Rules for Great Results

If you have made a decision to change your current eating habits, the 21-day kick start eating challenge is a great place to start. In only 3 weeks or 21 days, you will be on to a healthy eating path. To be clear, this challenge is not about micro-managing food intake.

Before you start, **_always consult a knowledgeable health professional about your diet or whether you should be following any particular eating/diet strategy._**

The challenge is simple - break any rule, start again at Day 1. The pages following the rules are for recording your progress during the challenge.

The 7 Rules for the 21-Day Kick Start Eating Challenge

Rule 1: Eat breakfast every morning.
Make time for breakfast. Smoothies are a great way to get daily servings of fruits and protein in the morning.

Rule 2: Eliminate refined sugar and replace with whole foods.
A few helpful hints:

- Avoid foods from boxes.
- Eat foods with a short list of ingredients.
- Avoid foods with ingredients you cannot pronounce.
- Avoid most processed foods.
- The only exception to this rule is for foods consumed during and immediately following a workout (within 45 minutes).

Rule 3: Drink more water.
A few helpful hints:

- For a hot beverage, green tea is a great option.
- Avoid juices - especially fruit juice blends or cocktails.
- Drink less alcohol. Calories from alcohol are considered empty calories and serve no nutritional purpose in the body.

Rule 4: Eat smaller meals every 2-3 hours.
A few other specifics to keep in mind:

- Consume the same daily volume of food, but in more frequent, smaller meals. Research has shown smaller meals increase metabolic rate and also ensure a steady insulin levels.
- Eat a high quality source of protein with every meal. Boiled eggs and

canned fish are convenient choices.

- Eat vegetables and fruits often and preferably with every meal. Lean toward eating more vegetables.

Rule 5: Reduce carbohydrate intake from grains and starchy sources.

Work on reducing carbohydrate intake from grains and try to eat more carbohydrates from vegetables and fruits. Eat as many different colours as possible when it comes to fruits and vegetables.

Rule 6: If you believe it is not a good food choice, then DON'T eat it.

Rule 7: Eat enough healthy fats (25-35% of the total daily intake).

Strive to eat healthy fats sources:

- Vegetables, such as avocados and olives, are good sources of unsaturated fats.

- Nuts contain high amounts of monounsaturated fats which have been shown to protect against cardiovascular disease. Certain peanut butter also contains healthy fats.

- Fish is rich in unsaturated fats and contain omega 3 fatty acids. Fish can be a great substitute to meats such as beef and pork (high saturated fats).

- Olive and canola oils are rich in unsaturated fats and great substitutes for butter while cooking.

LASTLY - The "Reward Meal"

Once each week, for a period limited to 60 minutes, eat whatever you want guilt free. Make sure you record the day of this meal so as not to have more than 3 during the challenge.

Credit must go to Terminal City Training for inspiring the basis of the challenge. They also credit John Berardi (www.johnberardi.com) and Dave Tate (www.elitefts.com) for inspiring many of the guidelines incorporated into this challenge.

This is where you would set your goal for the day for each area. Use appendix A to calculate how close you came to meeting the goal.

Date:_____

Nutrition Record

Goal:_____

(Protein _____% Carbs:_____ % Fat _____%)

*See **Appendix A** for formula to calculate total daily Calories

Meals	Cholesterol	Protein (grams)	Carbs (grams)	Fats (grams)	Trans
Meal #1 (Time _____)					
Meal #2 (Time _____)					
Meal #3 (Time _____)					
Meal #4 (Time _____)					
Meal #5 (Time _____)					
Totals grams (calculate total daily calories in Appendix A)		❶	❷	❸	

This is where you can keep track of everything that enters your mouth and when!

Note: You are able to keep track of the amount of cholesterol and trans fats too for each meal.

Vitamins / Medications / Additional Supplements

Take the total grams and use in Appendix A

Water (8oz): ☐☐☐☐☐☐☐☐☐☐

Keep track of your all your vitamins, medications and other supplements not included elsewhere.

Keep track of your water intake per day. Recommended is 8 x 8oz servings per day (there is space for 10).

Goal:_____

(Protein:_____% Carbs:_____ % Fat:_____%)

*See **Appendix A** for formula to calculate total daily Calories.

Date:_____

Nutrition Record - DAY 1

Meals	Chole sterol	Protein (grams)	Carbs (grams)	Fats (grams)	Trans
Meal #1 (Time: _____)					
Meal #2 (Time: _____)					
Meal #3 (Time: _____)					
Meal #4 (Time: _____)					
Meal #5 (Time: _____)					
Totals grams (calculate total daily calories in Appendix A)		❶	❷	❸	

Vitamins / Medications / Additional Supplements

Water (8oz): ☐☐☐☐☐☐☐☐☐☐

Date:_____

Goal:_____

Nutrition Record - DAY 2

(Protein:_____% Carbs:_____% Fat:_____%)

*See **Appendix A** for formula to calculate total daily Calories.

Meals	Chole sterol	Protein (grams)	Carbs (grams)	Fats (grams)	Trans
Meal #1 (Time: _____)					
Meal #2 (Time: _____)					
Meal #3 (Time: _____)					
Meal #4 (Time: _____)					
Meal #5 (Time: _____)					
Totals grams (calculate total daily calories in Appendix A)		❶	❷	❸	

Vitamins / Medications / Additional Supplements

Water (8oz): ☐ ☐ ☐ ☐ ☐ ☐ ☐ ☐ ☐

Goal:_____

(Protein:_____% Carbs:_____ % Fat:_____%)

*See **Appendix A** for formula to calculate total daily Calories.

Date:_____

Nutrition Record - DAY 3

Meals	Cholesterol	Protein (grams)	Carbs (grams)	Fats (grams)	Trans
Meal #1 (Time: _____)					
Meal #2 (Time: _____)					
Meal #3 (Time: _____)					
Meal #4 (Time: _____)					
Meal #5 (Time: _____)					
Totals grams (calculate total daily calories in Appendix A)		❶	❷	❸	

Vitamins / Medications / Additional Supplements

Water (8oz): ☐☐☐☐☐☐☐☐☐☐

Date:_____

Nutrition Record - DAY 4

Goal:_____

(Protein:_____% Carbs:_____% Fat:_____%)

*See **Appendix A** for formula to calculate total daily Calories.

Meals	Chole sterol	Protein (grams)	Carbs (grams)	Fats (grams)	Trans
Meal #1 (Time: _____)					
Meal #2 (Time: _____)					
Meal #3 (Time: _____)					
Meal #4 (Time: _____)					
Meal #5 (Time: _____)					
Totals grams (calculate total daily calories in Appendix A)		❶	❷	❸	

Vitamins / Medications / Additional Supplements

Water (8oz): ☐☐☐☐☐☐☐☐☐☐

Goal:_____

(Protein:_____% Carbs:_____ % Fat:_____%)

*See **Appendix A** for formula to calculate total daily Calories.

Date:_____

Nutrition Record - DAY 5

Meals	Chole sterol	Protein (grams)	Carbs (grams)	Fats (grams)	Trans
Meal #1 (Time: _____)					
Meal #2 (Time: _____)					
Meal #3 (Time: _____)					
Meal #4 (Time: _____)					
Meal #5 (Time: _____)					
Totals grams (calculate total daily calories in Appendix A)		❶	❷	❸	

Vitamins / Medications / Additional Supplements

Water (8oz): ☐ ☐ ☐ ☐ ☐ ☐ ☐ ☐ ☐ ☐

Date:_____

Nutrition Record - DAY 6

Goal:_____

(Protein:_____% Carbs:_____% Fat:_____%)

*See **Appendix A** for formula to calculate total daily Calories.

Meals	Chole sterol	Protein (grams)	Carbs (grams)	Fats (grams)	Trans
Meal #1 (Time: _____)					
Meal #2 (Time: _____)					
Meal #3 (Time: _____)					
Meal #4 (Time: _____)					
Meal #5 (Time: _____)					
Totals grams (calculate total daily calories in Appendix A)		❶	❷	❸	

Vitamins / Medications / Additional Supplements

Water (8oz): ☐☐☐☐☐☐☐☐☐☐

Goal:_____

(Protein:_____% Carbs:_____ % Fat:_____%)

*See **Appendix A** for formula to calculate total daily Calories.

Date:_____

Nutrition Record - DAY 7

Meals	Chole sterol	Protein (grams)	Carbs (grams)	Fats (grams)	Trans
Meal #1 (Time: _____)					
Meal #2 (Time: _____)					
Meal #3 (Time: _____)					
Meal #4 (Time: _____)					
Meal #5 (Time: _____)					
Totals grams (calculate total daily calories in Appendix A)		❶	❷	❸	

Vitamins / Medications / Additional Supplements

Water (8oz): ☐☐☐☐☐☐☐☐☐☐

Date:_____

Nutrition Record - DAY 8

Goal:_____

(Protein:_____% Carbs:_____ % Fat:_____%)

*See **Appendix A** for formula to calculate total daily Calories.

Meals	Cholesterol	Protein (grams)	Carbs (grams)	Fats (grams)	Trans
Meal #1 (Time: _____)					
Meal #2 (Time: _____)					
Meal #3 (Time: _____)					
Meal #4 (Time: _____)					
Meal #5 (Time: _____)					
Totals grams (calculate total daily calories in Appendix A)		❶	❷	❸	

Vitamins / Medications / Additional Supplements

Water (8oz): ☐☐☐☐☐☐☐☐☐☐

Goal:_____

(Protein:_____% Carbs:_____ % Fat:_____%)

*See **Appendix A** for formula to calculate total daily Calories.

Date:_____

Nutrition Record - DAY 9

Meals	Chole sterol	Protein (grams)	Carbs (grams)	Fats (grams)	Trans
Meal #1 (Time: _____)					
Meal #2 (Time: _____)					
Meal #3 (Time: _____)					
Meal #4 (Time: _____)					
Meal #5 (Time: _____)					
Totals grams (calculate total daily calories in Appendix A)		❶	❷	❸	

Vitamins / Medications / Additional Supplements

Water (8oz): ☐☐☐☐☐☐☐☐☐☐

Date:_____ Goal:_____

Nutrition Record - DAY 10

(Protein:_____% Carbs:_____ % Fat:_____%)

*See **Appendix A** for formula to calculate total daily Calories.

Meals	Chole sterol	Protein (grams)	Carbs (grams)	Fats (grams)	Trans
Meal #1 (Time:_____)					
Meal #2 (Time:_____)					
Meal #3 (Time:_____)					
Meal #4 (Time:_____)					
Meal #5 (Time:_____)					
Totals grams (calculate total daily calories in Appendix A)		❶	❷	❸	

Vitamins / Medications / Additional Supplements

Water (8oz): ☐☐☐☐☐☐☐☐☐☐

Goal:_____

(Protein:_____% Carbs:_____ % Fat:_____%)

*See **Appendix A** for formula to calculate total daily Calories.

Date:_____

Nutrition Record - DAY 11

Meals	Chole sterol	Protein (grams)	Carbs (grams)	Fats (grams)	Trans
Meal #1 (Time: _____)					
Meal #2 (Time: _____)					
Meal #3 (Time: _____)					
Meal #4 (Time: _____)					
Meal #5 (Time: _____)					
Totals grams (calculate total daily calories in Appendix A)		❶	❷	❸	

Vitamins / Medications / Additional Supplements

Water (8oz): ☐☐☐☐☐☐☐☐☐☐

Date:_____

Goal:_____

Nutrition Record - DAY 12

(Protein:_____% Carbs:_____ % Fat:_____%)

*See **Appendix A** for formula to calculate total daily Calories.

Meals	Chole sterol	Protein (grams)	Carbs (grams)	Fats (grams)	Trans
Meal #1 (Time: _____)					
Meal #2 (Time: _____)					
Meal #3 (Time: _____)					
Meal #4 (Time: _____)					
Meal #5 (Time: _____)					
Totals grams (calculate total daily calories in Appendix A)		❶	❷	❸	

Vitamins / Medications / Additional Supplements

Water (8oz): ☐☐☐☐☐☐☐☐☐☐

Goal:_____

(Protein:_____% Carbs:_____% Fat:_____%)

*See **Appendix A** for formula to calculate total daily Calories.

Date:_____

Nutrition Record - DAY 13

Meals	Chole sterol	Protein (grams)	Carbs (grams)	Fats (grams)	Trans
Meal #1 (Time: _____)					
Meal #2 (Time: _____)					
Meal #3 (Time: _____)					
Meal #4 (Time: _____)					
Meal #5 (Time: _____)					
Totals grams (calculate total daily calories in Appendix A)		❶	❷	❸	

Vitamins / Medications / Additional Supplements

Water (8oz): ☐☐☐☐☐☐☐☐☐☐

Date:_____

Nutrition Record - DAY 14

Goal:_____

(Protein:_____% Carbs:_____ % Fat:_____%)

*See **Appendix A** for formula to calculate total daily Calories.

Meals	Cholesterol	Protein (grams)	Carbs (grams)	Fats (grams)	Trans
Meal #1 (Time: _____)					
Meal #2 (Time: _____)					
Meal #3 (Time: _____)					
Meal #4 (Time: _____)					
Meal #5 (Time: _____)					
Totals grams (calculate total daily calories in Appendix A)		❶	❷	❸	

Vitamins / Medications / Additional Supplements

Water (8oz): ☐☐☐☐☐☐☐☐☐☐

Goal:_____

(Protein:_____% Carbs:_____ % Fat:_____%)

*See **Appendix A** for formula to calculate total daily Calories.

Date:_____

Nutrition Record - DAY 15

Meals	Chole sterol	Protein (grams)	Carbs (grams)	Fats (grams)	Trans
Meal #1 (Time: _____)					
Meal #2 (Time: _____)					
Meal #3 (Time: _____)					
Meal #4 (Time: _____)					
Meal #5 (Time: _____)					
Totals grams (calculate total daily calories in Appendix A)		❶	❷	❸	

Vitamins / Medications / Additional Supplements

Water (8oz): ☐☐☐☐☐☐☐☐☐☐

Date:_____

Nutrition Record - DAY 16

Goal:_____

(Protein:_____% Carbs:_____ % Fat:_____%)

*See **Appendix A** for formula to calculate total daily Calories.

Meals	Chole sterol	Protein (grams)	Carbs (grams)	Fats (grams)	Trans
Meal #1 (Time: _____)					
Meal #2 (Time: _____)					
Meal #3 (Time: _____)					
Meal #4 (Time: _____)					
Meal #5 (Time: _____)					
Totals grams (calculate total daily calories in Appendix A)		❶	❷	❸	

Vitamins / Medications / Additional Supplements

Water (8oz): ☐☐☐☐☐☐☐☐☐☐

Goal:_____

(Protein:_____% Carbs:_____% Fat:_____%)

*See **Appendix A** for formula to calculate total daily Calories.

Date:_____

Nutrition Record - DAY 17

Meals	Chole sterol	Protein (grams)	Carbs (grams)	Fats (grams)	Trans
Meal #1 (Time: _____)					
Meal #2 (Time: _____)					
Meal #3 (Time: _____)					
Meal #4 (Time: _____)					
Meal #5 (Time: _____)					
Totals grams (calculate total daily calories in Appendix A)		❶	❷	❸	

Vitamins / Medications / Additional Supplements

Water (8oz): ☐☐☐☐☐☐☐☐☐☐

Date:_____

Nutrition Record - DAY 18

Goal:_____

(Protein:_____% Carbs:_____ % Fat:_____%)

*See **Appendix A** for formula to calculate total daily Calories.

Meals	Chole sterol	Protein (grams)	Carbs (grams)	Fats (grams)	Trans
Meal #1 (Time: _____)					
Meal #2 (Time: _____)					
Meal #3 (Time: _____)					
Meal #4 (Time: _____)					
Meal #5 (Time: _____)					
Totals grams (calculate total daily calories in Appendix A)		❶	❷	❸	

Vitamins / Medications / Additional Supplements

Water (8oz): ☐☐☐☐☐☐☐☐☐

Goal:_____

(Protein:_____% Carbs:_____ % Fat:_____%)

*See **Appendix A** for formula to calculate total daily Calories.

Date:_____

Nutrition Record - DAY 19

Meals	Chole sterol	Protein (grams)	Carbs (grams)	Fats (grams)	Trans
Meal #1 (Time: _____)					
Meal #2 (Time: _____)					
Meal #3 (Time: _____)					
Meal #4 (Time: _____)					
Meal #5 (Time: _____)					
Totals grams (calculate total daily calories in Appendix A)		❶	❷	❸	

Vitamins / Medications / Additional Supplements

Water (8oz): ☐☐☐☐☐☐☐☐☐☐

Date:_____

Goal:_____

Nutrition Record - DAY 20

(Protein:_____% Carbs:_____ % Fat:_____%)

*See **Appendix A** for formula to calculate total daily Calories.

Meals	Chole sterol	Protein (grams)	Carbs (grams)	Fats (grams)	Trans
Meal #1 (Time: _____)					
Meal #2 (Time: _____)					
Meal #3 (Time: _____)					
Meal #4 (Time: _____)					
Meal #5 (Time: _____)					
Totals grams (calculate total daily calories in Appendix A)		❶	❷	❸	

Vitamins / Medications / Additional Supplements

Water (8oz): ☐☐☐☐☐☐☐☐☐☐

Goal:_____

(Protein:_____% Carbs:_____% Fat:_____%)

*See **Appendix A** for formula to calculate total daily Calories.

Date:_____

Nutrition Record - DAY 21

Meals	Chole sterol	Protein (grams)	Carbs (grams)	Fats (grams)	Trans
Meal #1 (Time: _____)					
Meal #2 (Time: _____)					
Meal #3 (Time: _____)					
Meal #4 (Time: _____)					
Meal #5 (Time: _____)					
Totals grams (calculate total daily calories in Appendix A)		❶	❷	❸	

Vitamins / Medications / Additional Supplements

Water (8oz): ☐ ☐ ☐ ☐ ☐ ☐ ☐ ☐ ☐ ☐

Date:_____

Nutrition Record - Bonus Day

Goal:_____

(Protein:_____% Carbs:_____ % Fat:_____%)

*See **Appendix A** for formula to calculate total daily Calories.

Meals	Chole sterol	Protein (grams)	Carbs (grams)	Fats (grams)	Trans
Meal #1 (Time: _____)					
Meal #2 (Time: _____)					
Meal #3 (Time: _____)					
Meal #4 (Time: _____)					
Meal #5 (Time: _____)					
Totals grams (calculate total daily calories in Appendix A)		❶	❷	❸	

Vitamins / Medications / Additional Supplements

Water (8oz): ☐☐☐☐☐☐☐☐☐☐

My Nutrition Log

21 Day Challenge #2

Date:_____

Goal:_____

Nutrition Record - DAY 1

(Protein:_____% Carbs:_____ % Fat:_____%)

*See **Appendix A** for formula to calculate total daily Calories.

Meals	Chole sterol	Protein (grams)	Carbs (grams)	Fats (grams)	Trans
Meal #1 (Time: _____)					
Meal #2 (Time: _____)					
Meal #3 (Time: _____)					
Meal #4 (Time: _____)					
Meal #5 (Time: _____)					
Totals grams (calculate total daily calories in Appendix A)		❶	❷	❸	

Vitamins / Medications / Additional Supplements

Water (8oz): ☐☐☐☐☐☐☐☐☐☐

Goal:_____

(Protein:_____% Carbs:_____ % Fat:_____%)

*See **Appendix A** for formula to calculate total daily Calories.

Date:_____

Nutrition Record - DAY 2

Meals	Chole sterol	Protein (grams)	Carbs (grams)	Fats (grams)	Trans
Meal #1 (Time: _____)					
Meal #2 (Time: _____)					
Meal #3 (Time: _____)					
Meal #4 (Time: _____)					
Meal #5 (Time: _____)					
Totals grams (calculate total daily calories in Appendix A)		❶	❷	❸	

Vitamins / Medications / Additional Supplements

Water (8oz): ☐☐☐☐☐☐☐☐☐☐

Date:_____

Nutrition Record - DAY 3

Goal:_____

(Protein:_____% Carbs:_____ % Fat:_____%)

*See **Appendix A** for formula to calculate total daily Calories.

Meals	Chole sterol	Protein (grams)	Carbs (grams)	Fats (grams)	Trans
Meal #1 (Time: _____)					
Meal #2 (Time: _____)					
Meal #3 (Time: _____)					
Meal #4 (Time: _____)					
Meal #5 (Time: _____)					
Totals grams (calculate total daily calories in Appendix A)		❶	❷	❸	

Vitamins / Medications / Additional Supplements

Water (8oz): ☐☐☐☐☐☐☐☐☐☐

Goal:_____

(Protein:_____% Carbs:_____ % Fat:_____%)

*See **Appendix A** for formula to calculate total daily Calories.

Date:_____

Nutrition Record - DAY 4

Meals	Chole sterol	Protein (grams)	Carbs (grams)	Fats (grams)	Trans
Meal #1 (Time: _____)					
Meal #2 (Time: _____)					
Meal #3 (Time: _____)					
Meal #4 (Time: _____)					
Meal #5 (Time: _____)					
Totals grams (calculate total daily calories in Appendix A)		❶	❷	❸	

Vitamins / Medications / Additional Supplements

Water (8oz): ☐☐☐☐☐☐☐☐☐☐

Date:_____

Nutrition Record - DAY 5

Goal:_____

(Protein:_____% Carbs:_____% Fat:_____%)

*See **Appendix A** for formula to calculate total daily Calories.

Meals	Chole sterol	Protein (grams)	Carbs (grams)	Fats (grams)	Trans
Meal #1 (Time:_____)					
Meal #2 (Time:_____)					
Meal #3 (Time:_____)					
Meal #4 (Time:_____)					
Meal #5 (Time:_____)					
Totals grams (calculate total daily calories in Appendix A)		❶	❷	❸	

Vitamins / Medications / Additional Supplements

Water (8oz): ☐☐☐☐☐☐☐☐☐☐

Goal:_____

(Protein:_____% Carbs:_____ % Fat:_____%)

*See **Appendix A** for formula to calculate total daily Calories.

Date:_____

Nutrition Record - DAY 6

Meals	Chole sterol	Protein (grams)	Carbs (grams)	Fats (grams)	Trans
Meal #1 (Time: _____)					
Meal #2 (Time: _____)					
Meal #3 (Time: _____)					
Meal #4 (Time: _____)					
Meal #5 (Time: _____)					
Totals grams (calculate total daily calories in Appendix A)		❶	❷	❸	

Vitamins / Medications / Additional Supplements

Water (8oz): ☐☐☐☐☐☐☐☐☐☐

Date:_____

Nutrition Record - DAY 7

Goal:_____

(Protein:_____% Carbs:_____ % Fat:_____%)

*See **Appendix A** for formula to calculate total daily Calories.

Meals	Chole sterol	Protein (grams)	Carbs (grams)	Fats (grams)	Trans
Meal #1 (Time:_____)					
Meal #2 (Time:_____)					
Meal #3 (Time:_____)					
Meal #4 (Time:_____)					
Meal #5 (Time:_____)					
Totals grams (calculate total daily calories in Appendix A)		❶	❷	❸	

Vitamins / Medications / Additional Supplements

Water (8oz): ☐☐☐☐☐☐☐☐☐☐

Goal:_____

(Protein:_____% Carbs:_____% Fat:_____%)

*See **Appendix A** for formula to calculate total daily Calories.

Date:_____

Nutrition Record - DAY 8

Meals	Chole sterol	Protein (grams)	Carbs (grams)	Fats (grams)	Trans
Meal #1 (Time: _____)					
Meal #2 (Time: _____)					
Meal #3 (Time: _____)					
Meal #4 (Time: _____)					
Meal #5 (Time: _____)					
Totals grams (calculate total daily calories in Appendix A)		❶	❷	❸	

Vitamins / Medications / Additional Supplements

Water (8oz): ☐☐☐☐☐☐☐☐☐☐

Date:_____ Goal:_____

Nutrition Record - DAY 9

(Protein:_____% Carbs:_____ % Fat:_____%)

*See **Appendix A** for formula to calculate total daily Calories.

Meals	Chole sterol	Protein (grams)	Carbs (grams)	Fats (grams)	Trans
Meal #1 (Time:_____)					
Meal #2 (Time:_____)					
Meal #3 (Time:_____)					
Meal #4 (Time:_____)					
Meal #5 (Time:_____)					
Totals grams (calculate total daily calories in Appendix A)		❶	❷	❸	

Vitamins / Medications / Additional Supplements

Water (8oz): ☐☐☐☐☐☐☐☐☐

Goal:_____

(Protein:_____% Carbs:_____% Fat:_____%)

*See **Appendix A** for formula to calculate total daily Calories.

Date:_____

Nutrition Record - DAY 10

Meals	Cholesterol	Protein (grams)	Carbs (grams)	Fats (grams)	Trans
Meal #1 (Time: _____)					
Meal #2 (Time: _____)					
Meal #3 (Time: _____)					
Meal #4 (Time: _____)					
Meal #5 (Time: _____)					
Totals grams (calculate total daily calories in Appendix A)		❶	❷	❸	

Vitamins / Medications / Additional Supplements

Water (8oz): ☐☐☐☐☐☐☐☐☐☐

Date:_____

Goal:_____

Nutrition Record - DAY 11

(Protein:_____% Carbs:_____% Fat:_____%)

*See **Appendix A** for formula to calculate total daily Calories.

Meals	Chole sterol	Protein (grams)	Carbs (grams)	Fats (grams)	Trans
Meal #1 (Time: _____)					
Meal #2 (Time: _____)					
Meal #3 (Time: _____)					
Meal #4 (Time: _____)					
Meal #5 (Time: _____)					
Totals grams (calculate total daily calories in Appendix A)		❶	❷	❸	

Vitamins / Medications / Additional Supplements

Water (8oz): ☐☐☐☐☐☐☐☐☐☐

Goal:_____

(Protein:_____% Carbs:_____% Fat:_____%)

*See **Appendix A** for formula to calculate total daily Calories.

Date:_____

Nutrition Record - DAY 12

Meals	Chole sterol	Protein (grams)	Carbs (grams)	Fats (grams)	Trans
Meal #1 (Time: _____)					
Meal #2 (Time: _____)					
Meal #3 (Time: _____)					
Meal #4 (Time: _____)					
Meal #5 (Time: _____)					
Totals grams (calculate total daily calories in Appendix A)		❶	❷	❸	

Vitamins / Medications / Additional Supplements

Water (8oz): ☐☐☐☐☐☐☐☐☐

Date:_____

Nutrition Record - DAY 13

Goal:_____

(Protein:_____% Carbs:_____ % Fat:_____%)

*See **Appendix A** for formula to calculate total daily Calories.

Meals	Chole sterol	Protein (grams)	Carbs (grams)	Fats (grams)	Trans
Meal #1 (Time: _____)					
Meal #2 (Time: _____)					
Meal #3 (Time: _____)					
Meal #4 (Time: _____)					
Meal #5 (Time: _____)					
Totals grams (calculate total daily calories in Appendix A)		❶	❷	❸	

Vitamins / Medications / Additional Supplements

Water (8oz): ☐☐☐☐☐☐☐☐☐☐

Goal:_____

(Protein:_____% Carbs:_____ % Fat:_____%)

*See **Appendix A** for formula to calculate total daily Calories.

Date:_____

Nutrition Record - DAY 14

Meals	Chole sterol	Protein (grams)	Carbs (grams)	Fats (grams)	Trans
Meal #1 (Time: _____)					
Meal #2 (Time: _____)					
Meal #3 (Time: _____)					
Meal #4 (Time: _____)					
Meal #5 (Time: _____)					
Totals grams (calculate total daily calories in Appendix A)		❶	❷	❸	

Vitamins / Medications / Additional Supplements

Water (8oz): ☐☐☐☐☐☐☐☐☐☐

Date:_____

Goal:_____

Nutrition Record - DAY 15

(Protein:_____% Carbs:_____% Fat:_____%)

*See **Appendix A** for formula to calculate total daily Calories.

Meals	Chole sterol	Protein (grams)	Carbs (grams)	Fats (grams)	Trans
Meal #1 (Time: _____)					
Meal #2 (Time: _____)					
Meal #3 (Time: _____)					
Meal #4 (Time: _____)					
Meal #5 (Time: _____)					
Totals grams (calculate total daily calories in Appendix A)		❶	❷	❸	

Vitamins / Medications / Additional Supplements

Water (8oz): ☐☐☐☐☐☐☐☐☐☐

Goal:_____

(Protein:_____% Carbs:_____ % Fat:_____%)

*See **Appendix A** for formula to calculate total daily Calories.

Date:_____

Nutrition Record - DAY 16

Meals	Chole sterol	Protein (grams)	Carbs (grams)	Fats (grams)	Trans
Meal #1 (Time: _____)					
Meal #2 (Time: _____)					
Meal #3 (Time: _____)					
Meal #4 (Time: _____)					
Meal #5 (Time: _____)					
Totals grams (calculate total daily calories in Appendix A)		❶	❷	❸	

Vitamins / Medications / Additional Supplements

Water (8oz): ☐☐☐☐☐☐☐☐☐☐

Date:_____ Goal:_____

Nutrition Record - DAY 17

(Protein:_____% Carbs:_____% Fat:_____%)

*See **Appendix A** for formula to calculate total daily Calories.

Meals	Chole sterol	Protein (grams)	Carbs (grams)	Fats (grams)	Trans
Meal #1 (Time: _____)					
Meal #2 (Time: _____)					
Meal #3 (Time: _____)					
Meal #4 (Time: _____)					
Meal #5 (Time: _____)					
Totals grams (calculate total daily calories in Appendix A)		❶	❷	❸	

Vitamins / Medications / Additional Supplements

Water (8oz): ☐☐☐☐☐☐☐☐☐☐

Goal:_____

(Protein:_____% Carbs:_____% Fat:_____%)

*See **Appendix A** for formula to calculate total daily Calories.

Date:_____

Nutrition Record - DAY 18

Meals	Cholesterol	Protein (grams)	Carbs (grams)	Fats (grams)	Trans
Meal #1 (Time: _____)					
Meal #2 (Time: _____)					
Meal #3 (Time: _____)					
Meal #4 (Time: _____)					
Meal #5 (Time: _____)					
Totals grams (calculate total daily calories in Appendix A)		❶	❷	❸	

Vitamins / Medications / Additional Supplements

Water (8oz): ☐☐☐☐☐☐☐☐☐☐

Date:_____

Goal:_____

Nutrition Record - DAY 19

(Protein:_____% Carbs:_____% Fat:_____%)

*See **Appendix A** for formula to calculate total daily Calories.

Meals	Cholesterol	Protein (grams)	Carbs (grams)	Fats (grams)	Trans
Meal #1 (Time: _____)					
Meal #2 (Time: _____)					
Meal #3 (Time: _____)					
Meal #4 (Time: _____)					
Meal #5 (Time: _____)					
Totals grams (calculate total daily calories in Appendix A)		❶	❷	❸	

Vitamins / Medications / Additional Supplements

Water (8oz): ☐☐☐☐☐☐☐☐☐☐

Goal:_____

(Protein:_____% Carbs:_____ % Fat:_____%)

*See **Appendix A** for formula to calculate total daily Calories.

Date:_____

Nutrition Record - DAY 20

Meals	Chole sterol	Protein (grams)	Carbs (grams)	Fats (grams)	Trans
Meal #1 (Time: _____)					
Meal #2 (Time: _____)					
Meal #3 (Time: _____)					
Meal #4 (Time: _____)					
Meal #5 (Time: _____)					
Totals grams (calculate total daily calories in Appendix A)		❶	❷	❸	

Vitamins / Medications / Additional Supplements

Water (8oz): ☐☐☐☐☐☐☐☐☐☐

Date:_____

Goal:_____

Nutrition Record - DAY 21

(Protein:_____% Carbs:_____% Fat:_____%)

*See **Appendix A** for formula to calculate total daily Calories.

Meals	Cholesterol	Protein (grams)	Carbs (grams)	Fats (grams)	Trans
Meal #1 (Time: _____)					
Meal #2 (Time: _____)					
Meal #3 (Time: _____)					
Meal #4 (Time: _____)					
Meal #5 (Time: _____)					
Totals grams (calculate total daily calories in Appendix A)		❶	❷	❸	

Vitamins / Medications / Additional Supplements

Water (8oz): ☐☐☐☐☐☐☐☐☐☐

Goal:_____

(Protein:_____% Carbs:_____% Fat:_____%)

*See **Appendix A** for formula to calculate total daily Calories.

Date:_____

Nutrition Record - Extra Day

Meals	Chole sterol	Protein (grams)	Carbs (grams)	Fats (grams)	Trans
Meal #1 (Time: _____)					
Meal #2 (Time: _____)					
Meal #3 (Time: _____)					
Meal #4 (Time: _____)					
Meal #5 (Time: _____)					
Totals grams (calculate total daily calories in Appendix A)		❶	❷	❸	

Vitamins / Medications / Additional Supplements

Water (8oz): ☐☐☐☐☐☐☐☐☐☐

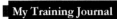

Appendix A

Nutrition Calculation

Date:_____   Calculation for Daily Nutrition

Step 1: Calculate Total Daily Calories for each Nutrient (❶❷❸ from page 189-233)

Grams of Protein ❶ [____] x **4** = ❹ [____]

Grams of Carbs ❷ [____] x **4** = ❺ [____]   ❹+❺+❻ = ❼ [____]

Grams of Fats ❸ [____] x **9** = ❻ [____]

Step 2: Calculate Total Percentage for Each Nutrient

Calories from Protein ❹ [____] ÷ ❼ [____] x **100** ❽ [____]

Calories from Carbs ❺ [____] ÷ ❼ [____] x **100** ❾ [____]

Calories from Fats ❻ [____] ÷ ❼ [____] x **100** ❿ [____]

Step 3: Comparison to Canada Food Guide Recommendations for Each Nutrient

Canada Food Guide Recommends: **Protein** ~**15** % VS ❽ [____]

Canada Food Guide Recommends: **Carbs** ~**55** % VS ❾ [____]

Canada Food Guide Recommends: **Fats** ~**30** % VS ❿ [____]

Date:_____   Calculation for Daily Nutrition

Step 1: Calculate Total Daily Calories for each Nutrient (❶❷❸ from page 189-233)

Grams of Protein ❶ [____] x **4** = ❹ [____]

Grams of Carbs ❷ [____] x **4** = ❺ [____]   ❹+❺+❻ = ❼ [____]

Grams of Fats ❸ [____] x **9** = ❻ [____]

Step 2: Calculate Total Percentage for Each Nutrient

Calories from Protein ❹ [____] ÷ ❼ [____] x **100** ❽ [____]

Calories from Carbs ❺ [____] ÷ ❼ [____] x **100** ❾ [____]

Calories from Fats ❻ [____] ÷ ❼ [____] x **100** ❿ [____]

Step 3: Comparison to Canada Food Guide Recommendations for Each Nutrient

Canada Food Guide Recommends: **Protein** ~**15** % VS ❽ [____]

Canada Food Guide Recommends: **Carbs** ~**55** % VS ❾ [____]

Canada Food Guide Recommends: **Fats** ~**30** % VS ❿ [____]

Date:_____ Calculation for Daily Nutrition

Step 1: Calculate Total Daily Calories for each Nutrient (❶❷❸ from page 189-233)

Grams of Protein ❶ [ ] x **4** = ❹ [ ]

Grams of Carbs ❷ [ ] x **4** = ❺ [ ]   ❹ + ❺ + ❻ = ❼ [ ]

Grams of Fats ❸ [ ] x **9** = ❻ [ ]

Step 2: Calculate Total Percentage for Each Nutrient

Calories from Protein ❹ [ ] ÷ ❼ [ ] x **100** ❽ [ ]

Calories from Carbs ❺ [ ] ÷ ❼ [ ] x **100** ❾ [ ]

Calories from Fats ❻ [ ] ÷ ❼ [ ] x **100** ❿ [ ]

Step 3: Comparison to Canada Food Guide Recommendations for Each Nutrient

Canada Food Guide Recommends: **Protein** ~**15** % vs ❽ [ ]

Canada Food Guide Recommends: **Carbs** ~**55** % vs ❾ [ ]

Canada Food Guide Recommends: **Fats** ~**30** % vs ❿ [ ]

Date:_____ Calculation for Daily Nutrition

Step 1: Calculate Total Daily Calories for each Nutrient (❶❷❸ from page 189-233)

Grams of Protein ❶ [ ] x **4** = ❹ [ ]

Grams of Carbs ❷ [ ] x **4** = ❺ [ ]   ❹ + ❺ + ❻ = ❼ [ ]

Grams of Fats ❸ [ ] x **9** = ❻ [ ]

Step 2: Calculate Total Percentage for Each Nutrient

Calories from Protein ❹ [ ] ÷ ❼ [ ] x **100** ❽ [ ]

Calories from Carbs ❺ [ ] ÷ ❼ [ ] x **100** ❾ [ ]

Calories from Fats ❻ [ ] ÷ ❼ [ ] x **100** ❿ [ ]

Step 3: Comparison to Canada Food Guide Recommendations for Each Nutrient

Canada Food Guide Recommends: **Protein** ~**15** % vs ❽ [ ]

Canada Food Guide Recommends: **Carbs** ~**55** % vs ❾ [ ]

Canada Food Guide Recommends: **Fats** ~**30** % vs ❿ [ ]

Date:_____ Calculation for Daily Nutrition

Step 1: Calculate <u>Total Daily Calories</u> for each Nutrient (❶❷❸ from page 189-233)

Grams of Protein ❶ [ ] x **4** = ❹ [ ]

Grams of Carbs ❷ [ ] x **4** = ❺ [ ] ❹+❺+❻ = ❼ [ ]

Grams of Fats ❸ [ ] x **9** = ❻ [ ]

Step 2: Calculate <u>Total Percentage</u> for Each Nutrient

Calories from Protein ❹ [ ] ÷ ❼ [ ] x **100** ❽ [ ]

Calories from Carbs ❺ [ ] ÷ ❼ [ ] x **100** ❾ [ ]

Calories from Fats ❻ [ ] ÷ ❼ [ ] x **100** ❿ [ ]

Step 3: Comparison to Canada Food Guide Recommendations for Each Nutrient

Canada Food Guide Recommends: **Protein** ~**15** % vs ❽ [ ]

Canada Food Guide Recommends: **Carbs** ~**55** % vs ❾ [ ]

Canada Food Guide Recommends: **Fats** ~**30** % vs ❿ [ ]

Date:_____ Calculation for Daily Nutrition

Step 1: Calculate <u>Total Daily Calories</u> for each Nutrient (❶❷❸ from page 189-233)

Grams of Protein ❶ [ ] x **4** = ❹ [ ]

Grams of Carbs ❷ [ ] x **4** = ❺ [ ] ❹+❺+❻ = ❼ [ ]

Grams of Fats ❸ [ ] x **9** = ❻ [ ]

Step 2: Calculate <u>Total Percentage</u> for Each Nutrient

Calories from Protein ❹ [ ] ÷ ❼ [ ] x **100** ❽ [ ]

Calories from Carbs ❺ [ ] ÷ ❼ [ ] x **100** ❾ [ ]

Calories from Fats ❻ [ ] ÷ ❼ [ ] x **100** ❿ [ ]

Step 3: Comparison to Canada Food Guide Recommendations for Each Nutrient

Canada Food Guide Recommends: **Protein** ~**15** % vs ❽ [ ]

Canada Food Guide Recommends: **Carbs** ~**55** % vs ❾ [ ]

Canada Food Guide Recommends: **Fats** ~**30** % vs ❿ [ ]

Date:_____   Calculation for Daily Nutrition

Step 1: Calculate Total Daily Calories for each Nutrient (❶❷❸ from page 189-233)

Grams of Protein	❶	x **4** =	❹		
Grams of Carbs	❷	x **4** =	❺	❹+❺+❻ =	❼
Grams of Fats	❸	x **9** =	❻		

Step 2: Calculate Total Percentage for Each Nutrient

Calories from Protein	❹	÷	❼	x **100**	❽
Calories from Carbs	❺	÷	❼	x **100**	❾
Calories from Fats	❻	÷	❼	x **100**	❿

Step 3: Comparison to Canada Food Guide Recommendations for Each Nutrient

Canada Food Guide Recommends: **Protein**	**~15 %**	VS	❽
Canada Food Guide Recommends: **Carbs**	**~55 %**	VS	❾
Canada Food Guide Recommends: **Fats**	**~30 %**	VS	❿

Date:_____   Calculation for Daily Nutrition

Step 1: Calculate Total Daily Calories for each Nutrient (❶❷❸ from page 189-233)

Grams of Protein	❶	x **4** =	❹		
Grams of Carbs	❷	x **4** =	❺	❹+❺+❻ =	❼
Grams of Fats	❸	x **9** =	❻		

Step 2: Calculate Total Percentage for Each Nutrient

Calories from Protein	❹	÷	❼	x **100**	❽
Calories from Carbs	❺	÷	❼	x **100**	❾
Calories from Fats	❻	÷	❼	x **100**	❿

Step 3: Comparison to Canada Food Guide Recommendations for Each Nutrient

Canada Food Guide Recommends: **Protein**	**~15 %**	VS	❽
Canada Food Guide Recommends: **Carbs**	**~55 %**	VS	❾
Canada Food Guide Recommends: **Fats**	**~30 %**	VS	❿

Date:_____   Calculation for Daily Nutrition

Step 1: Calculate Total Daily Calories for each Nutrient (❶❷❸ from page 189-233)

Grams of Protein ❶	$\times\,4 =$ ❹	
Grams of Carbs ❷	$\times\,4 =$ ❺	❹ + ❺ + ❻ = ❼
Grams of Fats ❸	$\times\,9 =$ ❻	

Step 2: Calculate Total Percentage for Each Nutrient

Calories from Protein ❹	÷ ❼	$\times\,100$	❽
Calories from Carbs ❺	÷ ❼	$\times\,100$	❾
Calories from Fats ❻	÷ ❼	$\times\,100$	❿

Step 3: Comparison to Canada Food Guide Recommendations for Each Nutrient

Canada Food Guide Recommends: **Protein**	~15 %	vs	❽
Canada Food Guide Recommends: **Carbs**	~55 %	vs	❾
Canada Food Guide Recommends: **Fats**	~30 %	vs	❿

Date:_____   Calculation for Daily Nutrition

Step 1: Calculate Total Daily Calories for each Nutrient (❶❷❸ from page 189-233)

Grams of Protein ❶	$\times\,4 =$ ❹	
Grams of Carbs ❷	$\times\,4 =$ ❺	❹ + ❺ + ❻ = ❼
Grams of Fats ❸	$\times\,9 =$ ❻	

Step 2: Calculate Total Percentage for Each Nutrient

Calories from Protein ❹	÷ ❼	$\times\,100$	❽
Calories from Carbs ❺	÷ ❼	$\times\,100$	❾
Calories from Fats ❻	÷ ❼	$\times\,100$	❿

Step 3: Comparison to Canada Food Guide Recommendations for Each Nutrient

Canada Food Guide Recommends: **Protein**	~15 %	vs	❽
Canada Food Guide Recommends: **Carbs**	~55 %	vs	❾
Canada Food Guide Recommends: **Fats**	~30 %	vs	❿

Appendix B

Before & After Pics

Date:_____

Goals & Photograph #1

Short term / long term goals and picture of physique.

Short Term Goals: **Date Due:**

1. _____ _____

2. _____ _____

3. _____ _____

Long Term Goals: **Date Due:**

1. _____ _____

2. _____ _____

Attach picture here

Date:_____

Short term / long term goals and picture of physique.

Goals & Photograph #2

Short Term Goals: **Date Due:**

1. _____   _____

2. _____   _____

3. _____   _____

Long Term Goals: **Date Due:**

1. _____   _____

2. _____   _____

Attach picture here

Date:_____

Goals & Photograph #3

Short term / long term goals and picture of physique.

Short Term Goals: **Date Due:**

1. _____   _____

2. _____   _____

3. _____   _____

Long Term Goals: **Date Due:**

1. _____   _____

2. _____   _____

Attach picture here

Appendix C

Sleep vs Workout Rating

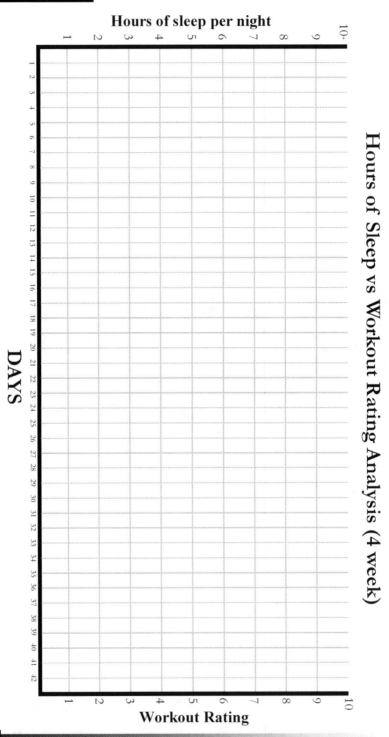

Hours of sleep per night

DAYS

Hours of Sleep vs Workout Rating Analysis (4 week)

Workout Rating

Appendix D

Health Assessment

Date:_____   Performed by:_____

Health & Fitness Assessment

Pre-Test Screening

	Reading 1	Reading 2
RHR (bpm)		
BP (mmhg)		
	BP <144/<94 & HR <100	
Weight		Kg/ lbs.
Height		Feet /Inches
BMI		Kg/m²

Girth Measurements

	Right	**Left**	**Around**
Upper Arm			
Chest			
Abdominal			
Waist			
Hip			
Thigh			
WHR			

Functional Movement Screen (FMS)

Overhead Squat	1	2	3	0
Hurdle Step (L)	1	2	3	0
Hurdle Step (R)	1	2	3	0
Inline Lunge (L)	1	2	3	0
Inline Lunge (R)	1	2	3	0
Shoulder (L)	1	2	3	0
Shoulder (R)	1	2	3	0
Shoulder (L)	YES	NO		
Shoulder (R)	YES	NO		
Push-Up	1	2	3	0
Cobra	YES	NO		
ASLR (L)	1	2	3	0
ASLR (R)	1	2	3	0
Anti-Rotatn (L)	1	2	3	0
Anti-Rotatn (R)	1	2	3	0
Child's Pose	YES	NO		
Total Score			<= 14 Poor	

Clips

	1	2	Average
Triceps			
Biceps			
Subscap			
Illiac Crest			
Umbilical			
Quads			
Med Calf			
Σ clips			
%BF			

Quantitative Measures

Grip	1	2	Average
Right hand	kg	kg	
Left hand	kg	kg	

Plank	<30 sec	31-59	60+

Power	1	2	3
Long Jump			
Vertical			

Cycle	Distance	
3 minute		km/miles
2 minute		km/miles

Performed by:_____

Date:_____

Health & Fitness Assessment

Pre-Test Screening

	Reading 1	Reading 2
RHR (bpm)		
BP (mmhg)		
	BP <144/<94 & HR <100	
Weight		Kg/ lbs.
Height		Feet /Inches
BMI		Kg/m²

Functional Movement Screen (FMS)

Overhead Squat	1	2	3	0
Hurdle Step (L)	1	2	3	0
Hurdle Step (R)	1	2	3	0
Inline Lunge (L)	1	2	3	0
Inline Lunge (R)	1	2	3	0
Shoulder (L)	1	2	3	0
Shoulder (R)	1	2	3	0
Shoulder (L)	YES	NO		
Shoulder (R)	YES	NO		
Push-Up	1	2	3	0
Cobra	YES	NO		
ASLR (L)	1	2	3	0
ASLR (R)	1	2	3	0
Anti-Rotatn (L)	1	2	3	0
Anti-Rotatn (R)	1	2	3	0
Child's Pose	YES	NO		
Total Score			<= 14 Poor	

Girth Measurements

	Right	**Left**	**Around**
Upper Arm			
Chest			
Abdominal			
Waist			
Hip			
Thigh			
WHR			

Clips

	1	2	Average
Triceps			
Biceps			
Subscap			
Illiac Crest			
Umbilical			
Quads			
Med Calf			
Σ clips			
%BF			

Quantitative Measures

Grip	1	2	Average
Right hand	kg	kg	
Left hand	kg	kg	
Plank	<30 sec	31-59	60+
Power	1	2	3
Long Jump			
Vertical			
Cycle	Distance		
3 minute			km/miles
2 minute			km/miles

Date:_____ Performed by:_____

Health & Fitness Assessment

Pre-Test Screening

	Reading 1	Reading 2
RHR (bpm)		
BP (mmhg)		
	BP <144/<94 & HR <100	
Weight		Kg/ lbs.
Height		Feet /Inches
BMI		Kg/m²

Girth Measurements

	Right	**Left**	**Around**
Upper Arm			
Chest			
Abdominal			
Waist			
Hip			
Thigh			
WHR			

Functional Movement Screen (FMS)

Overhead Squat	1	2	3	0
Hurdle Step (L)	1	2	3	0
Hurdle Step (R)	1	2	3	0
Inline Lunge (L)	1	2	3	0
Inline Lunge (R)	1	2	3	0
Shoulder (L)	1	2	3	0
Shoulder (R)	1	2	3	0
Shoulder (L)	YES	NO		
Shoulder (R)	YES	NO		
Push-Up	1	2	3	0
Cobra	YES	NO		
ASLR (L)	1	2	3	0
ASLR (R)	1	2	3	0
Anti-Rotatn (L)	1	2	3	0
Anti-Rotatn (R)	1	2	3	0
Child's Pose	YES	NO		
Total Score			<= 14 Poor	

Clips

	1	2	Average
Triceps			
Biceps			
Subscap			
Illiac Crest			
Umbilical			
Quads			
Med Calf			
Σ clips			
%BF			

Quantitative Measures

Grip	1	2	Average
Right hand	kg	kg	
Left hand	kg	kg	

Plank	<30 sec	31-59	60+

Power	1	2	3
Long Jump			
Vertical			

Cycle	Distance	
3 minute		km/miles
2 minute		km/miles

Appendix E

Sample Programs

Sample Training Programs

Go to:

vipfitness.ca/programs.shtml

For sample programs to help get you started or to provide ideas for a new approach!

Another book written by Aaron Tews:

Sample pages:

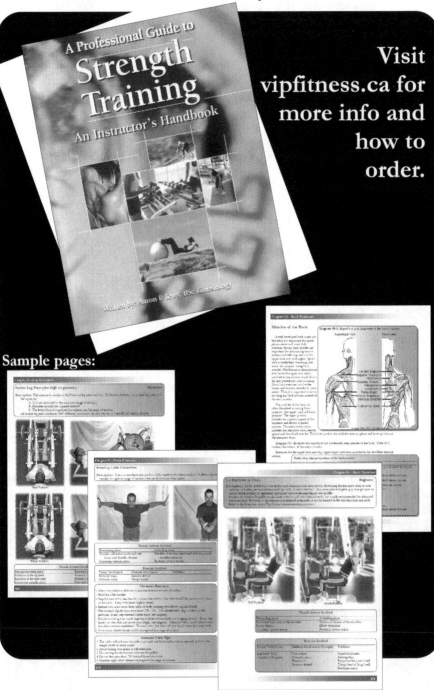